CONTENTS

SECOND EDITION

JUMPING INTO PLYOMETRICS

DONALD CHU, PhD

ATHER SPORTS INJURY CLINIC
CASTRO VALLEY, CALIFORNIA

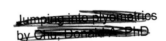
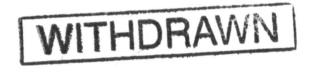

Library of Congress Cataloging-in-Publication Data

Chu, Donald A. (Donald Allen), 1940-
    Jumping into plyometrics / by Donald A. Chu. -- 2nd ed.
      p.   cm.
    Includes bibliographical references (p.   ) and index.
    ISBN 0-88011-846-6 (pbk.)
    1. Physical education and training.   2. Exercise.   I. Title.
  GV711.C54   1998
  613.7'11--dc21   98-17867
                                   CIP

ISBN: 0-88011-846-6

Acquisitions Editor: Martin Barnard; **Developmental Editor**: Laura Casey Mast; **Assistant Editor**: Cynthia McEntire; **Copyeditor**: Jim Burns; **Proofreader**: Kathy Bennett; **Indexer**: Nancy Ball; **Graphic Designer**: Nancy Rasmus; **Graphic Artist**: Sandra Meier; **Photo Editor**: Boyd LaFoon; **Cover Designer**: Jack Davis; **Photographer (cover)**: Tom Roberts; **Photographer (interior)**: Tom Roberts; **Illustrators**: Keith Blomberg, Joe Bellis; **Printer**: United Graphics

Human Kinetics books are available at special discounts for bulk purchase. Special editions or book excerpts can also be created to specification. For details, contact the Special Sales Manager at Human Kinetics.

Copies of this book are available at special discounts for bulk purchase for sales promotions, premiums, fund-raising, or educational use. Special editions or book excerpts can also be created to specifications. For details, contact the Special Sales Manager at Human Kinetics.

Printed in the United States of America   10 9

Human Kinetics
Web site: www.HumanKinetics.com

United States: Human Kinetics, P.O. Box 5076, Champaign, IL 61825-5076
800-747-4457
e-mail: humank@hkusa.com

Canada: Human Kinetics, 475 Devonshire Road, Unit 100, Windsor, ON N8Y 2L5
800-465-7301 (in Canada only)
e-mail: orders@hkcanada.com

Europe: Human Kinetics, 107 Bradford Road, Stanningley
Leeds LS28 6AT, United Kingdom
+44 (0) 113 255 5665
e-mail: hk@hkeurope.com

Australia: Human Kinetics, 57A Price Avenue, Lower Mitcham, South Australia 5062
08 8277 1555
e-mail: liahka@senet.com.au

New Zealand: Human Kinetics, P.O. Box 105-231, Auckland Central
09-523-3462
e-mail: hkp@ihug.co.nz

PREFACE

The evolution of performance enhancement in today's athletic world is truly amazing. Since *Jumping Into Plyometrics* was first published in 1992, there has been a virtual explosion in the number of trainers and coaches embracing plyometric training as an integral part of their athletes' development. Originating from track and field, this system of exercise has grown from mystery to commonplace. The end user's knowledge of these exercises has grown dramatically. Sports such as synchronized swimming, once far removed from the concept of power, credit plyometrics for raising the level of performance.

The second edition of *Jumping Into Plyometrics* is an update of plyometric knowledge. New and exciting drills to improve footwork and basic movement skills have been added. Drills extend from beginner to more advanced skills. Additional research supporting the inclusion of plyometrics in various sport training programs has also been added. Five new sports have been added to chapter 5, covering an even broader area. Athlete profiles highlight the performance edge some professional athletes have gained using plyometrics in their training programs.

Plyometric exercise merges the physical qualities of speed and strength to produce an athlete capable of running faster and jumping higher. Furthermore, the expansion of plyometrics to cover the multi-directional athlete provides greater variety and even more sport-specific options when designing a training program.

The body of knowledge concerning the effects of plyometric training on performance has been expanded. The ability to get the "biggest bang for your buck" in sport training is now available. Not only do plyometrics fit into the complete training program, a training program is not complete *without* plyometrics.

Plyometric training has undergone a considerable metamorphosis over the past few years. New ideas and innovative techniques will lead the reader into the second generation of plyometric training. The coach or trainer who understands the options and opportunities available through plyometric training will find new ways to train athletes. I wish you well in undertaking the *smart* way versus the *hard* way to work and train.

UNDERSTANDING PLYOMETRICS

This chapter describes the development of plyometric training and the methods by which athletes have experienced significant improvement in performance through using plyometrics. I cover the physiology of plyometrics along with the relationship of other fitness variables, such as flexibility and aerobic and anaerobic training, to plyometric training programs.

THE DEVELOPMENT OF PLYOMETRIC TRAINING

Plyometrics is the term now applied to exercises that have their roots in Europe, where they were first known simply as "jump training."

Interest in this jump training increased during the early 1970s as East European athletes emerged as powers on the world sport scene. As the Eastern bloc countries began to produce superior athletes in such sports as track and field, gymnastics, and weightlifting, the mystique of their success began to center on their training methods.

The actual term *plyometrics* was first coined in 1975 by Fred Wilt, one of America's more forward-thinking track and field coaches. Based on Latin origins, *plyo + metrics* is interpreted to mean "measurable increases." These seemingly exotic exercises were thought to be responsible for the rapid competitiveness and growing superiority of Eastern Europeans in track and field events.

Plyometrics rapidly became known to coaches and athletes as exercises or drills aimed at linking strength with speed of movement to produce power. Plyometric training became essential to athletes who jumped, lifted, or threw.

During the late 1970s and into the 1980s, those in other sports also began to see the applicability of these concepts to their own movement activities. Throughout the 1980s, coaches in sports such as volleyball, football, and weightlifting began to use plyometric exercises and drills to enhance their training programs. If there was any drawback to this enthusiasm, it lay with the lack of expertise that American coaches and athletes had in administering plyometric programs and a faulty belief that more must be better. Since these early growth years, however, practitioners have learned through applied research, as well as trial and error, to establish realistic expectations.

THE SCIENCE OF PLYOMETRIC TRAINING

The '90s have seen a great deal of effort expended on attempts to verify the effectiveness and safety of plyometrics. As might be expected, the results of these studies are mixed. Athletes of various sports and equally varied levels of conditioning have been compared to "untrained" athletes under all sorts of variables and conditions. The point that is missed in this research is that athletic development follows its own time curve. A 6-, 12-, or 24-week testing period can in no way reflect the longitudinal development that will occur throughout an athlete's overall career. For some, this time span may be a single season, for others, it may be up to 30 years of highly competitive activity.

Therefore, plyometric training should be considered in the context of the athlete's age, skill levels, injury history, and a myriad of other variables that comprise his or her athletic development. In this way through applied research practitioners can learn to establish realistic expectations.

HOW PLYOMETRICS WORKS

Plyometrics is defined as exercises that enable a muscle to reach maximum strength in as short a time as possible. This speed-strength ability is known as power. Although most coaches and athletes know that power is the name of the game, few have understood the mechanics necessary to develop it. To help you understand plyometrics, I'll review some of the important points of muscle physiology. This will serve to demonstrate the simple, yet complex, way in which plyometric training relates to better performance.

PHYSIOLOGY OF MUSCLES

Muscles, along with bones, provide for posture and movement in the human body. Muscles are our only musculoskeletal structures that can lengthen and shorten (figure 1.1). Unlike ligaments and tendons, the other supporting structures, muscles possess a unique ability to impart dynamic activity to the body. (Ligaments are tough, dense, fibrous tissues that attach bone to bone to provide both support and mobility. Tendons are the very fibrous structures that attach muscles to bones.)

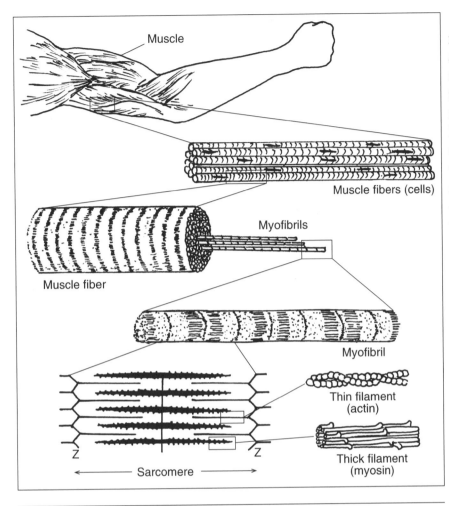

Figure 1.1 The structure of the muscle cell.

Two types of muscle fiber make up muscles: extrafusal and intrafusal. Extrafusal fibers contain myofibrils, the elements that contract, relax, and elongate muscles. Myofibrils are made up of several bands, and between the bands are units called sarcomeres. Sarcomeres contain myofilaments made up of the proteins actin and myosin. The myosin myofilaments have small projections, called cross-bridges, extending from them. Extrafusal fibers receive nerve impulses from the brain that cause a chemical reaction. This reaction eventually causes the cross-bridges in the myosin to collapse and allows the actin and myosin myofilaments to slide over one another and the muscle fiber to shorten, or contract.

Intrafusal fibers, also called muscle spindles, lie parallel to the extrafusal fibers. Muscle spindles are the main stretch receptors in muscle. When a muscle is stretched, the muscle spindles receive a message from the brain that initiates a stretch reflex.

Muscles derive information from the central nervous system, or brain. This information travels through the spinal cord out into the peripheral nervous system, which extends from the spinal cord, between the vertebrae, and ultimately to every muscle in the body. Among the messages reaching the muscles are those governing the length of each muscle at any point, the expected tension necessary for maintaining posture and initiating or stopping movement. An unbelievable amount of information is processed in each second.

TYPES OF MUSCLE CONTRACTIONS

In sport activity the athlete has to be concerned with three modes of muscle contraction: eccentric, isometric, and concentric.

Eccentric contractions, which occur when the muscle lengthens under tension, are used to decelerate the body. In a runner's stride, for example, the impact of contacting the ground on a single foot requires the body's center of gravity to drop rapidly. The runner does not collapse at this moment because the leg muscles can contract and control this lowering motion.

Midstride, the body comes to a complete halt and an *isometric* contraction occurs, a static position in which there is no muscle shortening visible to the observer. In sport activities, this contraction occurs in the brief instant between the eccentric contraction and the subsequent concentric contraction, in which the muscle fibers pull together and shorten. This concentric contraction then results in acceleration of the limb segments in running.

USING KNOWLEDGE OF MUSCLE PHYSIOLOGY IN TRAINING

Eccentric (lengthening) muscle contractions are rapidly followed by concentric (shortening) contractions in many sport skills. Whenever a long jumper makes contact with the takeoff board, for example, there is an absorption of the shock of landing marked by slight flexion of the hip, knee, and ankle, followed by a rapid extension of the takeoff foot and leg as the jumper leaves the board.

Or think about the basketball player who drives for the slam dunk. As the player takes the last step toward the basket, the supporting leg must take the full body weight and stop the horizontal inertia of the run-up. This "loads" the leg by rapidly forcing its muscles to stretch and undergo a rapid eccentric contraction. Nerves firing information to the muscle then cause a concentric contraction. These muscle responses occur with no conscious thought on the part of the player, but without them the player's knee would buckle and he would collapse to the floor.

Another way of thinking about these muscle actions is to imagine a spring. In the case of the basketball player, the run-up puts pressure on the takeoff leg, compressing the coils of the spring. The energy stored within the spring is then released as the athlete leaves the floor.

Research from studies examining great jumpers and sprinters or other athletes who rely on the speed and strength capability of muscles shows that they do not spend much time on the ground. These elite athletes have learned that energy is stored during the eccentric phase of muscle contraction and is partially recovered during the concentric contraction. However, the potential energy developed in this process can be lost (in the form of heat generation) if the eccentric contraction is not immediately followed by a concentric contraction. This conversion from negative (eccentric) to positive (concentric) work was described in the European literature as the amortization phase. This coupling of the eccentric-concentric contraction takes place within hundredths of a second. Typically, great high jumpers are on the ground a mere 0.12 seconds!

An entire system of exercise—plyometrics—has arisen just to address the development of a shorter amortization phase. And, perhaps surprisingly, the length of the amortization phase is largely dependent on learning. Where strength and innate speed are important, an athlete can shorten the amortization phase by applying learning and skill training to a base of strength development.

PHYSIOLOGY OF PLYOMETRICS

Because the term plyometrics is a later creation, much of the early related physiological research is described by other names. The term used by researchers in Italy, Sweden, and the Soviet Union for this type of muscle action was the *stretch-shortening cycle*.

The physiological research supporting plyometrics, or the stretch-shortening cycle of muscle tissue, has been reviewed by many authors. The consensus of opinion cites the importance of two factors: (a) the serial elastic components of muscle, which include the tendons and the cross-bridging characteristics of the actin and myosin that make up the muscle fibers; and (b) the sensors in the muscle spindles (proprioceptors) that play the role of presetting muscle tension and relaying sensory input related to rapid muscle stretching for activation of the "stretch reflex."

Muscle elasticity is an important factor in understanding how the stretch-shortening cycle can produce more power than a simple concentric muscle contraction. As illustrated in the earlier descriptions of jumping, the muscles can briefly store the tension developed by rapid stretching so that they possess a sort of potential elastic energy. For an analogy, consider a rubber band—whenever you stretch it, there exists the potential for a rapid return to its original length.

The stretch reflex is another mechanism integral to the stretch-shortening cycle. A common example of the stretch reflex is the knee jerk experienced when the quadriceps tendon is tapped with a rubber mallet. The tapping causes the quadriceps tendon to stretch. That stretching is sensed by the quadriceps muscle, which contracts in response.

The stretch, or myotatic, reflex responds to the rate at which a muscle is stretched and is among the fastest in the human body. The reason for this is the direct connection from sensory receptors in the muscle to cells in the spinal cord and back to the muscle fibers responsible for contraction. Other reflexes are slower than the stretch reflex because they must be transmitted through several different channels (interneurons) and to the central nervous system (brain) before a reaction is elicited.

The importance of this minimal delay in the stretch reflex is that muscle undergoes a contraction faster during a stretch-shortening cycle than in any other method of contraction. A voluntary or thought-out response to muscle stretch would be too late to be of use to an athlete jumping, running, or throwing.

Besides response time, response strength is a consideration when determining how plyometrics relates to sport performance. Although the response time of the stretch reflex remains about the same even after training, training changes the strength of the response in terms of muscle contraction. The faster a muscle is stretched or lengthened, the greater its concentric force after the stretch. The result is a more forceful movement for overcoming the inertia of an object, whether it is the individual's own body weight (as in running or jumping) or an external object (a shot put, a blocking bag, an opponent, etc.).

POWER TRAINING

The quest for optimal power training has led to the development of various training methods. Traditionally, heavy resistance training techniques have been used to improve strength and, subsequently, performance. These techniques have typically used weights of 80 to 90 percent of one-repetition maximum for repetitions of four to six in number. More current thought combines a variety of training modalities, including plyometrics, dynamic weightlifting, and combinations of these, to enhance explosive power.

The research has indicated that heavy lifting and plyometrics as methods of training have effectively improved power output. This led to thinking that a combination of both systems could result in even greater improvements. This has proven to be so, particularly in the area of vertical jumping.

The question that remained was whether lifting for maximal power output, as opposed to maximum strength, could be of benefit to the athlete. Maximum power lifting occurs when the lifts are made more dynamic in nature. An example of this type of lifting is the exercise known as "jump squats." In this exercise the athlete utilizes a load of approximately 30 to 60 percent of one-rep maximum to perform the particular lifts. The result is a faster, more powerful movement through the full range of motion. The idea is do "maximal power training" in that the amount of resistive load maximizes the mechanical power output of the exercise. The 5-5-5 squat embodies this principle. This exercise is performed with a lighter than maximal load for five parallel squats, followed by five squats done "quickly," and five squat jumps. The quick squats are to be performed as if the athlete were dropping out from under the resistance and utilizing a "catch" position at the bottom of the movement. The squat jump obviously requires the athlete to explode through the full range of motion up to and through the point where the feet actually leave contact with the ground.

Extensive research has demonstrated that maximal strength levels can be improved by using lighter weights while doing highly accelerated movements in both the upper and lower extremities. This type of training is known in the East European literature as *complex* training. Using maximal power output training and plyometrics in an integrated fashion can lead to rapid increases in strength, although the intensity of this type of training would be too stressful for long-term training (greater than a 12-week cycle). However, it can be applied when short periods of training are desired or available and it can be used as preparation for competition in a fully periodized training year.

FLEXIBILITY

Anyone undertaking a plyometric training program should have a reasonable amount of flexibility. Static stretching, which increases flexibility, uses passive techniques to change the structures of ligaments, tendons, and muscles. The muscle is put into a stretched position and held for 6 to 15 seconds (sometimes more); this is then repeated three times.

Ballistic stretching involves elongating a muscle to its normal length, bouncing gently against the end of the range 6 to 12 times, then repeating this action three times. Although research has shown static stretching techniques to be as effective as and possibly safer than ballistic stretching, ballistic stretching is still a valuable means of increasing range of motion.

Each method has its benefits, and in light of the principles of eliciting the stretch reflex and the serial elastic components of muscle to perform jumping activities, it might behoove the athlete to "prime" the mechanism by doing controlled ballistic stretching.

Aerobic Training

Aerobic capacity is a valuable component of most fitness programs. However, plyometric training, by the nature of the energy systems being utilized, is not intended to develop aerobic capacity. Plyometric training is strictly anaerobic (without oxygen) in nature and utilizes the creatine phosphate energy system, allowing maximum energy to be stored in the muscle before a single explosive act, using maximum power, is performed. It is a program that exploits a quality of movement compatible with single repetition, maximal efforts. Recovery should be complete between each repetition of the exercise and between each set of repetitions. If sufficient recovery is not allowed, then the activity may move toward being aerobic, but quality of movement and explosiveness are sure to suffer.

Summary

1. There are three types of muscular contractions:

- Eccentric
- Isometric
- Concentric

2. For an exercise to be truly plyometric, it must be a movement preceded by an eccentric contraction. This results not only in stimulating the proprioceptors sensitive to rapid stretch, but also in loading the serial elastic components (the tendons and cross-bridges between muscle fibers) with a tension force from which they can rebound.

3. A reasonable amount of flexibility is important when beginning a plyometric training program. Two types of stretching can be used to develop flexibility:

- Static
- Ballistic

4. Plyometric training is not intended to develop aerobic capacity and therefore requires complete recovery between reps and sets.

5. Research has shown the method of using training loads of 30 to 60 percent of 1RM in weightlifting to be an effective means of developing maximal power output. Combined with plyometrics, this form of training can be effective, time efficient, and safe.

THE BASICS OF PLYOMETRIC TRAINING

Now that you understand the inner workings of the muscular system and how they can be manipulated to create faster movements, let's turn our attention to exercises and drills that will create this change.

This chapter categorizes various plyometric exercises and explains the effects that can be achieved by using them. Plyometric training can take many forms, including jump training for the lower extremities and medicine ball exercises for the upper extremities. The user of plyometrics should understand not only how to do the exercises, but also how to implement and modify a program and use it to its best advantage.

WARM-UP: SUBMAXIMAL PLYOMETRIC DRILLS

One of the basic tenets of all exercise programs is that major efforts of training should be preceded by lower-level activities. These "warm-up" activities can take several different forms, and can be "general" or "specific" in nature. The exercises of choice when using plyometric drills should be specific or related to the larger efforts. These exercises are not classified as true plyometrics because they require less voluntary effort, focus, and concentration to complete. However, they are used to develop fundamental movement skills and therefore are helpful in establishing motor patterns that are going to directly carry over to speed development and jumping ability.

Before we get into the actual classification of jump training exercises let's take a look at some of the activities that fit into the warm-up or submaximal plyometrics category. Keep in mind that all of these drills are performed not as conditioning drills, but as skill enhancement drills aimed at teaching or rehearsing certain motor patterns. Therefore, they are performed over distances of 10 to 20 meters, with a relatively long recovery between exercises. A good rule of thumb to use in this situation is to have the athlete perform the drill in one direction, and walk back in the other. This allows for recovery as well as mental rehearsal for the next repetition.

If several exercises (8 to 12) are grouped in "sets" of three repetitions they can truly become a warm-up activity in that they will almost surely raise the athlete's core temperature and insure activities that will help in motor development. Administrating a group of athletes is made easier in that the individuals can be placed in groups according to ability and need for instruction.

MARCHING DRILLS

These drills are intended to mimic running movements (figure 2.1). They are intended to break down the act of running into its components. This allows the coach to stress component parts such as posture, joint angles, range of motion, foot placement, and other biomechanical features that are often overlooked when the whole activity is simply asked to be performed. Several Canadian track and field coaches (Mach, MacFarlane, Biancani) were early proponents of the use of these types of drills to enhance proper hip, thigh, and leg actions preparatory to running.

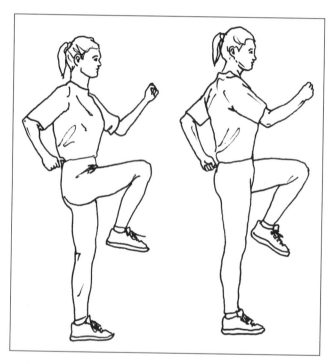

Figure 2.1   Marching drills.

JOGGING DRILLS

There are many variations of jogging that can be used to emphasize speed development because they can be modified to be plyometric in nature. The simple act of jogging on the toes with special emphasis on quick ground reaction by not letting the heel touch the ground can be a mini-plyometric activity (figure 2.2a). Jogging with the legs straight and limiting knee flexion will prepare the athlete to expect a sharp impact when performing maximal-effort plyometric drills (figure 2.2b). Special effects can be achieved by such drills as "butt-kickers" which emphasize knee flexion and bringing the heel to the buttocks (figure 2.2c); these can be extremely useful when the coach begins to work on the "recovery" phase of sprinting. This movement teaches the athlete that the shortest lever they have to swing forward will speed up their ability to cycle or turn over the legs during running. Heel recovery is an essential ingredient in absolute speed development.

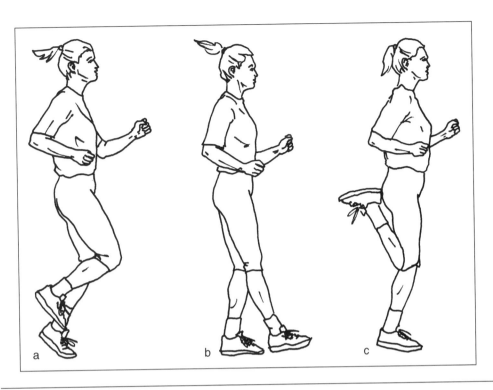

Figure 2.2 Jogging drills.

SKIPPING DRILLS

Synchronization of limb movements is basic to normal motor development. So-called reciprocal movements occur between the legs and arms in running. Generally speaking, efficient running requires a runner to move his left arm forward as the right leg comes forward, then switch limb movements to the opposite side of the body as he moves forward. This reciprocal motion is fundamental to the development of the athlete. Skipping activities require an exaggerated form of this reciprocal motion which is often lost if not practiced. Because of the requirements to perform reciprocal limb movements and the emphasis on quick takeoff and landing during skipping, this activity is ideal as a submaximal plyometric activity that can be used to warm up the athlete and prepare him for more complex skills (figure 2.3).

FOOTWORK DRILLS

There is a complete section on submaximal footwork drills in chapter 4 as developed and presented by John Frappier (1995) in his "Acceleration Training" program. However, there are drills which require hip movement and quick changes of direction that can also be used as warm-up drills. Drills such as the shuttle drills, multidirectional side shuffle drills, and "drop" step drills all fit under this heading (figure 2.4).

LUNGING DRILLS

These drills are taken from the basic exercise movement known as the "lunge" (figure 2.5). When used as submaximal drills, these exercises can take many

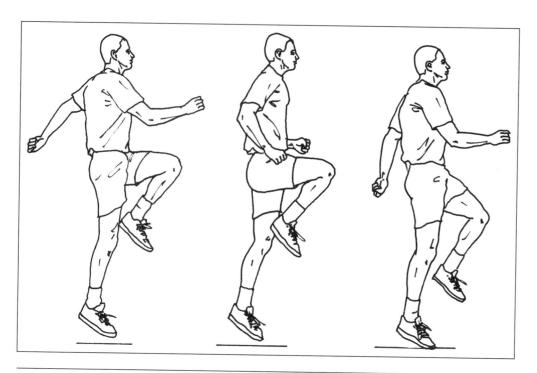

Figure 2.3   Skipping drills.

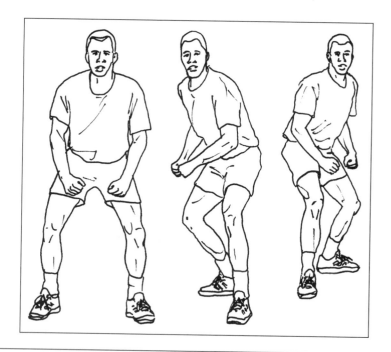

Figure 2.4   Footwork drills.

forms, and are known as forward lunges, side, crossover, multidirectional, reverse, and walking lunges. They can, and should always, be used as preparation before doing long amplitude jumps. These drills can be extremely useful in developing basic strength in the upper hip and thigh areas when used with simple body weight.

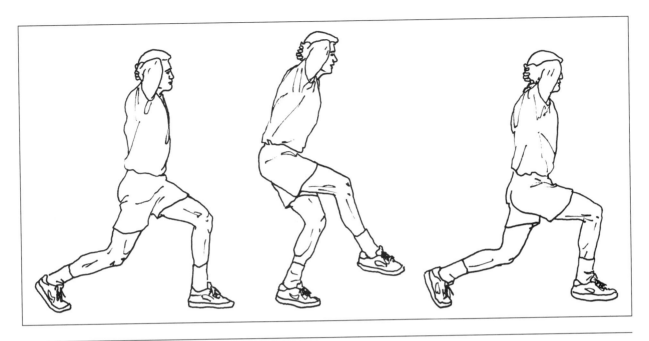

Figure 2.5 Lunging drills.

ALTERNATIVE MOVEMENT DRILLS

These drills include those movements not previously classified. Each activity is aimed at a specific area of the body with a special effect in mind when doing the drill.

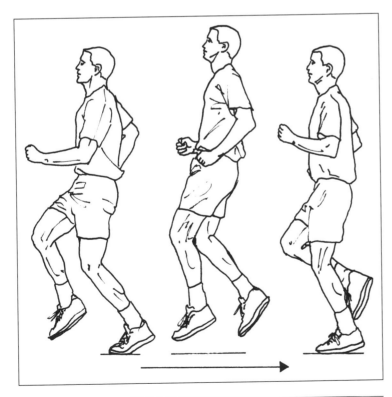

Figure 2.6 Alternate movement drill: backward running.

BACKWARD RUNNING

Hamstring and hip extension are never to be overlooked in the development of the athlete and in the prevention of injuries. Backward running has a particular way of strengthening the hamstrings in preparation for the tremendous eccentric forces applied to this area when running straight ahead (figure 2.6). Many practitioners of rehabilitation advocate backpedaling as an important rehabilitation exercise for the athlete following injury.

CARIOCA

This movement is probably as familiar to football coaches as the three-point stance. It has long been used to improve hip rotation and foot placement. The upper body is held relatively stationary as the player

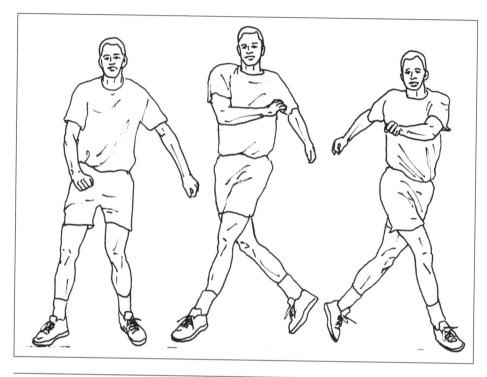

Figure 2.7 Alternate movement drill: carioca.

travels down a line sideways, then the feet are switched from a crossover position to a reversed position in rapid fashion (figure 2.7).

CLASSIFICATION OF JUMPS

Early jump training exercises were classified according to the relative demands they placed on the athlete. But all of them can be progressive in nature, with a range of low to high intensity in each type of exercise. The classifications I use in this book are similar to those used by the Europeans. You should note, however, that early writings from the Soviet Union classified hops and jumps on the basis of distance rather than type of exercise. *Hops* were exercises performed for distances less than 30 meters, while *jumps* were performed for distances greater than 30 meters. This classification can become confusing, so in this book the words *hop* and *jump* are used interchangeably.

JUMPS-IN-PLACE

A jump-in-place is exactly that: a jump completed by landing in the same spot where the jump started. These exercises are relatively low intensity, yet they provide the stimulus for developing a shorter amortization phase by requiring the athlete to rebound quickly from each jump. Jumps-in-place are done one after another, with a short amortization phase. Jumps in this category have been called "jumps-on-a-spot" and "multiple response jumps" by other authors.

STANDING JUMPS

A standing jump stresses single maximal effort, either horizontal or vertical. The exercise may be repeated several times, but full recovery should be allowed between each effort. The start of the exercise is generally a "ready position" with both feet shoulder-width apart. These have been called "single response" efforts in some literature.

MULTIPLE HOPS AND JUMPS

Multiple hops and jumps combine the skills developed by jumps-in-place and standing jumps. They require maximal effort but are done one after another. These exercises can be done alone or with a barrier. An advanced form of multiple hops and jumps is the box drill. Multiple hops and jumps should be done for distances of less than 30 meters.

BOUNDING

Bounding exercises exaggerate normal running stride to stress a specific aspect of the stride cycle. They are used to improve stride length and frequency, and typically are performed for distances greater than 30 meters.

BOX DRILLS

Box drills combine multiple hops and jumps with depth jumps. They can be low in intensity or extremely stressful, depending on the height of the boxes used. They incorporate both horizontal and vertical components for successful completion.

DEPTH JUMPS

Depth jumps use the athlete's body weight and gravity to exert force against the ground. Depth jumps are performed by stepping out from a box and dropping to the ground, then attempting to jump back up to the height of the box. Because depth jumps are of a prescribed intensity, one should never jump from the top of the box, as this adds height and increases the landing stress. Rather, one should attempt to step out into space before dropping to the ground. Controlling the height dropped helps not only to accurately measure intensity but also to reduce overuse problems. Upon making contact with the ground, the athlete directs the body up as fast as possible. The key to performing this exercise and decreasing the amortization phase is to stress the "touch and go" action off the ground.

RESEARCH ON DEPTH JUMPS

There seems to have been a fascination with studying the depth jump. The early Soviet research concluded that depth jumps were an effective means of increasing athletes' speed and strength capabilities. Verhoshanski (1969) proclaimed 0.8 meters as the ideal height for achieving maximum speed in switching from the eccentric to the concentric phase of the stretch-shortening cycle and 1.1 meters for developing maximal dynamic strength. He also recommended no more than 40 jumps in a single workout, performed no more than twice a week. Recovery between sets was facilitated by light jogging and calisthenics.

A later study by Verhoshanski and Tatyan (1983) comparing three groups of athletes showed that depth jumps were more effective than weight training, the jump-and-reach, or horizontal hops for developing speed and strength capabilities. Other researchers, such as Adams (1984), Bosco and Komi (1979), and Asmussen and Bonde-Peterson (1974) have sought the optimal height for depth jumps. Over a dozen studies conducted in the United States and Europe have served only to confuse the issue.

Research conducted in the United States since the late 1970s has shown that depth jumps generally increase athletes' abilities to jump higher in test situations. Any conflicts in the research about the effects of depth jumps are probably due to the many experimental designs that have been used. Recent efforts by Holcomb et al. (1996), Gehri et al. (n.d.), and Holcomb et al. (1996) have examined the differences between training with the depth jump (DJ) versus the countermovement jump (CMJ). The mechanical distinction between these two activities is that the CMJ is simply flexing the hips, knees, and ankles, allowing for a rapid descent of the body's center of gravity before using concentric muscle activity to jump vertically, while the DJ requires the use of body weight to eccentrically load the muscles via a vertical drop from a prescribed height. This activity requires the athlete to time the drop and be prepared to reverse the descent (eccentric to concentric muscle action) at the time the stimulus is perceived (when the feet make contact with the ground). Although statistical significance was revealed only amongst the groups tested on vertical jump with countermovement, raw data indicates that the group trained plyometrically using DJ improved in both peak power and vertical jump height more than any of the other groups when using either the countermovement or static starting position on vertical jump tasks.

There is no doubt that the learning factor is part of the success in effectively utilizing the depth jump in a training program. For achieving maximum results there are timing factors that must be trained as well as positioning factors, showing why the coaching of technique in the performance of these exercises needs to be learned and adhered to. Young et al. (1995) found that instructions given to subjects play a significant role in the type of jumping ability that is developed. Three groups were instructed to emphasize different aspects of the vertical jump, i.e., overall height achieved, time spent on the ground, and both maximum height and minimum ground contact. A fourth group stressed training with the countermovement type jump. The study showed that by using different instructions and giving feedback, clear differences in the characteristics of the jump were accomplished. When the objective of the jump was absolute height, regardless of time spent on the ground, depth jumps and countermovement jumps were similar. However, when contact time was considered, depth jump technique was considerably altered and resulted in low correlation between the tasks. Since the absolute height between DJ and

CMJ are unrelated when ground contact time is reduced, it is important to train as specifically for the sport task as possible.

The relative simplicity of performing the depth jump has made it an easy task to study. Investigators have tried to relate depth jumps to improvements in start speed, acceleration, and absolute speed in running and jumping but have tended to ignore the more elusive role of horizontal jump training (standing jumps, multiple jumps, and bounding). But because running and jumping involve both horizontal and vertical components, it seems to make sense that both horizontal and vertical jump training would contribute to improvements in both activities.

DETERMINING DEPTH JUMP HEIGHT

In practical terms, the task of determining a proper depth jump height centers on the ability to achieve maximal elevation of the body's center of gravity after performing a depth jump. If the height is too great for the strength of the legs, then the legs spend too much time absorbing the impact of the landing and cannot reverse the eccentric loading quickly enough to take advantage of the serial elastic component of muscle and the stretch reflex phenomenon. The result is a slow jump dependent on strength and devoid of power. Coach and athlete should work to find the proper height, one that lets the athlete maximize the height jumped plus achieve the shortest amortization phase.

One method described by many authors for determining maximum depth jump height is outlined in the sidebar.

HOW TO DETERMINE MAXIMUM DEPTH JUMP HEIGHT

1. The athlete is measured as accurately as possible for a standing jump-and-reach. (See page 87 for instructions on how to do a standing jump-and-reach.)

2. The athlete performs a depth jump from an 18-inch box height, trying to attain the same standing jump-and-reach score.

3. If the athlete successfully executes this task, he or she may move to a higher box. The box height should be increased in 6-inch increments. Step 2 is repeated until the athlete fails to reach the standing jump-and-reach height. This then becomes the athlete's maximum height for depth jumps.

4. If the athlete cannot reach the standing jump-and-reach height from an 18-inch box, either the height of the box should be lowered or depth jumping abandoned for a time in favor of strength development. If the athlete cannot rebound from a basic height of 18 inches, he or she probably does not have the musculoskeletal readiness for depth jumping.

MECHANICS OF VERTICAL JUMPING

Vertical jumping is a component of most sport activities. It is often taken for granted that an athlete instinctually knows how to jump vertically. In actuality,

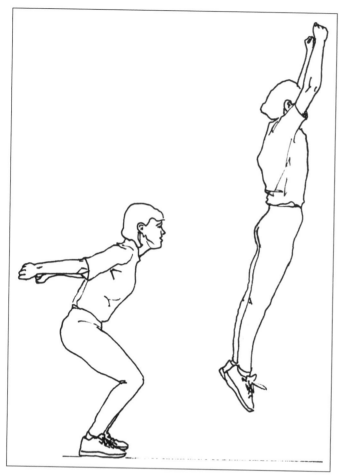

Figure 2.8 Maximum force development, arms back and straight.

jumping vertically is a skill that can and should be taught to athletes. If we examine the event a little more closely we find that the jump is preceded by a countermovement, in which the center of gravity (C of G) drops rapidly. This is seen as a flexing of the hips, knees, and ankles of the athlete. The trunk tilts slightly forward and the arms are pulled to a position behind the midline of the body. Prior to the vertical movement of the body, there is a rapid extension of the hips, knees, and ankles, which is largely the result of force developed by the arms and legs. The arms should be brought forward rapidly and allowed to travel to a position above and in front of the shoulders. The quick bend of the knees which lowers the C of G is accompanied by moving the arms into a position where the shoulders are extended and the arms are behind the athlete. This position of the arms allows the athlete to develop force which is directed into the ground as the arms come forward. Interestingly enough, once the arms pass the midline of the body they can no longer develop force that will help achieve overall height. Past this point they are only able to decelerate, and this allows the body to begin liftoff. Therefore, it is important to get the arms as far back and as straight as possible for maximum force development (figure 2.8). The more the arms bend at the elbow the faster they will come through, but the less they will contribute to overall force development. A practical view of this is to compare the arm swing of elite triple jumpers versus that of elite high jumpers. Where maximum force is important for the triple jumper, high jumpers using the Flop technique must rely more on arm speed to effectively carry out their technique.

Research by Everett Harman, PhD, et al. (1991) at the U.S. Army Research Institute of Environmental Medicine has shown that the countermovement is crucial to development of force and can contribute up to six percent of the total jump height. The arms can increase the overall jump height attained by as much as 21 percent. It was concluded that the arms developed their positive effect by exerting downward force on the body as they swung through in the early phase of the jump and kept the body in a position such that the quadriceps and gluteus muscles could exert force over a longer period of time. It was also concluded that since the countermovement did not contribute that significantly to jump height, many sport situations may not require a countermovement in order for the athlete to be effective. If speed of movement and reaction time is more crucial, such as in a volleyball block, the athlete may be just as effective by simply starting the jump with the knees bent. In other words, if an athlete does not need to attain maximum height a no-countermovement will clearly be the more effective.

Due to the arms' large contribution to overall jump height it appears that strengthening these areas through resistance training exercises would be an important component of all jump training programs. Some of the exercises seen as important in the development of the arms for jumping include the following:

1. Reverse Pull-Downs
2. Triceps Dips
3. Shoulder Swings
4. Straight Arm Lateral Pull-Downs
5. Seated Rows
6. Backward Medicine Ball Throws
7. Underhand Medicine Ball Throws

EQUIPMENT AND ENVIRONMENT

Plyometric training is quite versatile. It can be performed indoors or out—the basic requirements are adequate space and a yielding landing surface (with some give to prevent jarring the lower extremities with excessive force). Resilite wrestling mats, spring-loaded gymnastics or aerobics floors, and grass or synthetic playing fields are all possibilities for landing pads.

As far as space is concerned, it need simply be free of obstructions. Gym floors, large weight rooms, and outdoor fields are all suitable environments so long as the landing surface is appropriate.

A significant advantage to plyometric training is that it requires so little prefabricated equipment. The following represents the ultimate list of needed items.

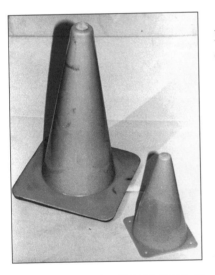

Figure 2.9   Plastic cones.

Plastic cones (figure 2.9) ranging in height from 8 to 24 inches serve as barriers over which to jump. The flexibility of cones makes them less likely to cause injuries if landed on.

Boxes do need to be specially constructed, but they are far from complex in their design. A variety of boxes, constructed of 3/4-inch plywood or a similar flexible yet durable wood, are needed. Boxes should range in height from 6 to 24 inches (with greater heights up to 42 inches only for elite athletes with strong weight training backgrounds). The boxes also need adequate landing (top) surfaces of at least 18 by 24 inches. To make nonslip landing surfaces, attach treads like those used on stairways, mix sand into the paint used to cover the boxes, or glue carpeting or rubberized flooring to the landing surfaces. Figure 2.10 shows a standard plyometric box.

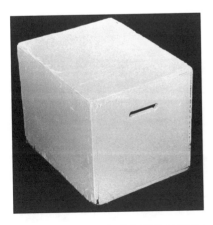

Figure 2.10   A standard plyometric box.

Numerous variations of the plyometric box have been developed over the years:

- Adjustable boxes (figure 2.11)—boxes that can be altered to accommodate the varying abilities of athletes.

- Storage boxes (figure 2.12)—boxes that can double as storage containers. (If one side is left open, the box needs to be constructed very sturdily on the remaining sides.)

- Special effects boxes (figure 2.13)—built to provide a special type of exercise stimulus. The most common of these is an angle box, which emphasizes the small muscles of the ankle and lower leg. The angle box is used to prevent ankle injuries by teaching athletes to learn to land on irregular surfaces. It is also useful in the rehabilitation of ankle and knee injuries.

In schools, physical education and athletic departments can often collaborate with industrial arts departments to build plyometric boxes. This is cost-effective and can promote a camaraderie between departments as students see their products being put to use.

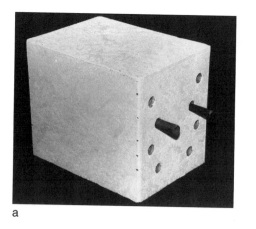
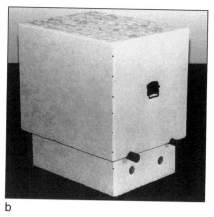

a
b

Figure 2.11 An adjustable plyometric box: (a) the base and (b) fully assembled.

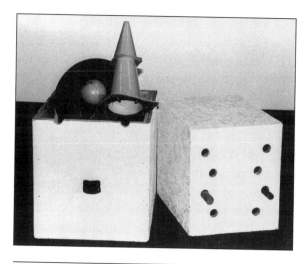

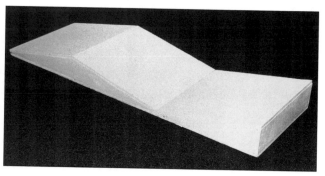

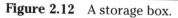

Figure 2.12 A storage box.

Figure 2.13 A special effects box (angled).

Most school physical education programs own hurdles and barriers. Hurdles, which are adjustable for degree of difficulty, do represent a hazard because of their rigid construction, and they should be used only by experienced plyometric exercisers (see figure 2.14).

Foam barriers (figure 2.15) are manufactured for gymnastics and tumbling. Barriers can also be constructed by scoring Styrofoam sheets on one side and then folding them to form soft triangular obstacles.

Barriers can also be formed simply by balancing a wooden dowel (1/2-inch diameter and 3 feet long) on top of two cones (figure 2.16).

Stairways, bleachers, and stadium steps are all usable for plyometric training, with one word of caution: Inspect them carefully to make sure they are safe for jumping. Concrete steps are undesirable for jumping because they are unyielding surfaces.

Weighted objects such as medicine balls (figure 2.17) are useful for upper body exercises and in combination with lower extremity training. They should be easily gripped, durable, and of varying weights to accommodate all strength levels.

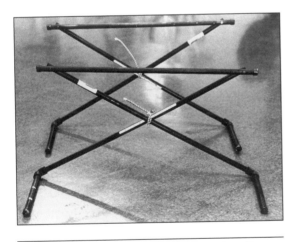

Figure 2.14   PVC pipe adjustable hurdles.

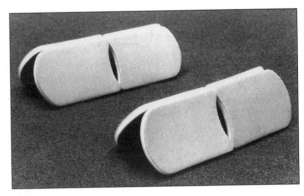

Figure 2.15   Foam barriers.

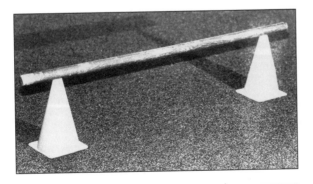

Figure 2.16   A cone-and-dowel barrier.

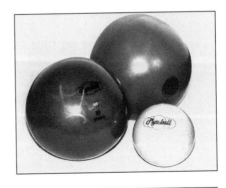

Figure 2.17   Medicine balls.

TRAINING CONSIDERATIONS

Plyometric training can be structured to individuals or to groups. Individual training requires exercisers to perform every task to the best of their ability (according to their level of development). It focuses on responsibility, concentration, and follow-through to complete the training session.

Group achievement can be structured so as to encompass, in addition to physical skills, social skills like communication, cooperation, trust, and immediate and long-term feedback in goal setting and achievement. Both individual and group sessions should take place in an environment that is positive in nature and emphasizes individual development.

There are several considerations in implementing a plyometric training program, whether for an individual or a group. The most important of these are common sense and experience. Programs must be prudently planned and administered. One of the major tasks is to conduct a needs analysis, taking into account the athlete's sport and the specific movements the athlete must perform to participate effectively. The needs analysis is covered in more depth in chapter 3. Other issues to consider are the athlete's age, experience, and athletic maturity.

The responsibility in initiating a plyometric program is enormous. The best coaches do not always win with their athletes, but they do make training an enjoyable, organized, and progressive activity that ultimately leads the athlete to higher levels of performance.

SEX

The myth that females must train differently than males still exists in some circles. But there is no reason that female athletes cannot perform plyometrics with the same degree of skill, proficiency, and intensity as males. The controlling factor of having a strength base is applicable to both sexes. Any athlete who chooses to ignore complementary strength training is headed for difficult times and perhaps injury. It is true that many female athletes are new to strength training and thus may not possess the requisite entry-level abilities. It is the responsibility of the coach and the athlete to upgrade this area of development before attempting plyometric training.

AGE

The simple factor of attention span is probably the major consideration in starting youngsters in plyometric training programs. Children will always run and jump as a part of play. But as adults we tend to take this element of play (known also as "fun"!) out of training programs by rigidly applying specific regimens.

YOUNG ATHLETES

Elementary school children can successfully do plyometric training as long as the coach does not call it plyometrics. Children of this age need images, such as animals in the forest jumping over streams and logs, to relate to. They can visualize and cognitively grasp the ease and skill with which a deer bounds through the woods. If movement patterns are placed in the proper context, children can attempt to express them in a "plyometric" fashion. In fact, hopscotch is a great early plyometric drill!

PUBESCENT ATHLETES

Young athletes can benefit more from direct training as they approach pubescence. They can begin to relate more to sport situations and see the correlation between what the coach asks them to do and their development in their sport.

Plyometrics for this group should always begin as gross motor activities of low intensity. They should be introduced into warm-ups and then added to sport-specific drills.

ADULT ATHLETES

As athletes approach the stage of individualization, they can begin to look at developing off-season and preseason training programs as preparation for performance. For most athletes this will be upon reaching high school, although in certain activities (ice skating, gymnastics, swimming, diving, dance, and track and field) the coach and the athlete may need to begin developing training cycles that use regimented plyometrics at an earlier age. This also depends on the athlete's level of competition.

TRAINING LEVEL

Two considerations regarding training level are important when structuring a plyometric training program: the intensity level of the exercise and the experience of the athlete. Plyometric training should be a progression of exercises and skilled movements that are considered to be elementary, intermediate, and advanced in scope. They should focus on improving the ballistic and reactive skills of the exerciser and are to be considered stressful. Drills should be evaluated for intensity before they are incorporated into a workout. Examples of low-, moderate-, and high-intensity drills may be found in chapter 4. Categorizing exercises by intensity helps both in choosing starting points for exercise and in developing program progression.

Another factor in program design is the training experience of the athlete. Though this may sound obvious, consider that one of the early European writings on jump training stated that athletes had to perform squats with 2.5 times their body weight before starting plyometrics—if every 150-pound athlete had to demonstrate squat strength of 375 pounds, there would be very few athletes doing plyometrics!

Practical experience has shown that many athletes benefit from plyometrics without demonstrating such leg strength. The exercise must be geared to the individual. An athlete who is barely past pubescence and is relatively unskilled should be considered a beginner. Beginners should be placed in a complementary resistance training program and should progress slowly and deliberately into a program of low-intensity plyometrics such as skipping drills, 8-inch cone hops, and box drills from 6 to 12 inches.

High school competitors who have been exposed to weight training programs can benefit from moderately intense plyometrics. And accomplished, mature, college-level athletes with strong weight training backgrounds should be able to perform ballistic-reactive exercises of high intensity with no undue problems. Once a classification of beginner, intermediate, or advanced has been generally determined, one can begin to plan a program.

ECCENTRIC STRENGTH

Eccentric strength, or the ability of a muscle to lengthen while under tension, is an important consideration for all athletes and is crucial for injured ones. Given that healthy limbs often have difficulty sustaining the impact placed on the body during practice and competition, it is essential that injured athletes returning to activity have some means of ensuring a safe and complete return.

Physical therapists and other rehabilitation specialists are beginning to recognize the importance of eccentric strength in rehabilitating musculo-skeletal injuries. Research has shown that eccentric strength is crucial to the return of injured athletes to their sports.

Eccentric strength is a precursor to success in plyometrics. Before an injured athlete can return to plyometric training there has to be an interval of training that focuses on the development of stability and eccentric strength in the lower extremities. Resistance training that isolates a single joint (open kinetic chain activities) and relegates it to performing single plane movements will not "rehabilitate" the athlete sufficiently to return her or him to activity. Simply put, you do not play the game sitting in a chair. Closed kinetic chain activities, which require the athlete to use the lower extremities in functional movement patterns involving the foot, ankle, knee, and hip have risen to the top of the list of effective rehabilitation exercises. Plyometric training also falls into the realm of closed kinetic chain activities.

Plyometric drills and skill activities can serve as functional tests to determine an injured athlete's readiness for return to play. The environment of competition places tremendous mental and physical stress on participants, and not being sure of one's physical ability is to risk a disastrous performance and, worse, reinjury. One recent study (Drez et al., 1987) cited single leg hops for a distance and timed single leg hops of six meters (about 20 feet) as a major determinant in the recovery of injuries to the anterior cruciate ligament in the knee. The ability to complete this task revealed a great deal about whether an athlete was truly ready to return to play. A below-normal score on these single leg hop tests indicated a knee at risk of giving way during sport activities. A passing score is determined by a symmetry score of 85 percent. The involved leg is tested twice and the average between the two trials is recorded. Then the noninvolved leg is tested in the same way. The scores of the noninvolved extremity are divided by the scores of the involved leg and multiplied by 100. This constitutes the symmetry index score, recorded as a percentage.

SPECIFICITY OF TRAINING

Plyometric training is very specific in nature but very broad in applicability. For the lower extremities, it is designed to train the athlete to develop either vertical or horizontal acceleration, and all movements in running and jumping are simply the exertion of some vertical or horizontal force against the ground. Even changes of direction fall into this category. Medicine ball exercises train the upper extremities and can also be used in combination with lower extremity training.

Specificity is a key concept, then, to keep in mind when planning a plyometric training program. The sport and the skill to be developed must be analyzed so proper exercises can be emphasized. To develop start speed from a crouch position, like an offensive lineman might assume, it doesn't make sense to spend a lot of time on depth jump skills, which develop vertical power. A more worthwhile exercise might be the standing long jump or double leg hops, which develop horizontal force.

Or perhaps the goal is to improve a basketball player's rebounding ability. Analyzing rebounding reveals that the skills needed are reacting quickly in a vertical motion and repeating jump height (because the first jump may not succeed in getting the rebound). This player, then, need not invest lots of time in jumps that emphasize horizontal abilities, such as double leg hops or bounds. Chapter 3 explains how to develop a program with these considerations in mind.

SUMMARY

1. There are six classifications of lower extremity plyometric exercises:

- Jumps-in-place
- Standing jumps
- Multiple hops and jumps
- Bounding
- Box drills
- Depth jumps

Medicine ball exercises train the upper extremities.

2. The following basic equipment is needed to conduct a plyometric training program:

- Cones
- Boxes
- Hurdles or barriers
- Stairs
- Medicine balls

3. The most important consideration in implementing and administering a plyometric training program is the athlete. Age, experience, and athletic maturity are all important criteria in establishing and modifying plyometric training.

4. Eccentric strength development is important for all athletes, and particularly so for injured athletes.

5. Plyometric training can be adapted to virtually every sport, and athletes should do exercises that help to enhance the movements they perform. By mimicking certain movements in plyometric training, athletes can decrease movement time and become more powerful.

Jim Grabb: Men's Doubles Tennis Player

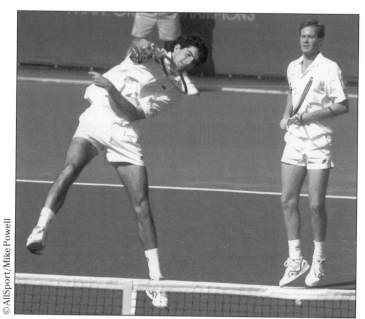

© AllSport/Mike Powell

Jim used plyometrics to make a successful return to the men's tour after shoulder surgery to repair the rotator cuff. He used medicine ball exercises to restore strength to his ground stroke. He also used several lower extremities exercises, such as cone hops, zigzag drills, and box jumps, to improve his speed and quickness.

One of the unique things Jim did was to count the number of shoulder contacts that he would incur during the course of a singles tennis match. Shoulder contacts were defined as the number of times he made contact with the tennis ball in any form of stroke. The number was a staggering 240 to 260 times during a five-set match. Therefore, we patterned his exercises to meet that particular demand. His medicine ball program might have looked like this (all exercises done with a 15-pound medicine ball unless otherwise indicated):

4 sets of 25 reps pull-over passes

2 sets of 20 reps lateral passes (both sides)

2 sets of 10 reps over-and-back lateral passes (both sides)

2 sets of 25 reps power drops from a 36-inch box with 20-pound ball

There were 270 throws in this one exercise session. Each session varied as to the type of exercise, but the intensity and the volume stayed relatively consistent. The only change came when speed of movement was the goal and then we changed to a lighter ball for faster sets.

In 1997, Jim and his doubles partner Wayne Black advanced to the quarterfinals at both the U.S. Open and at Wimbledon.

III

Designing a Plyometric Training Program

Now that you have a grasp of the basics, let's turn our attention to actually designing a plyometric training program. An art form as well as a science, this manipulation of variables can either create a champion or foster an "also-ran."

This chapter will cover the factors of plyometric training program design. It will discuss some of the concepts relevant to developing a basic, sport-specific, or advanced program.

Included are several sample training programs and the rationale behind creating them. Three sample programs deal with specific sports: synchronized swimming, baseball, and soccer. Two sample four week programs deal with improving vertical and linear jumping ability. Granted, four weeks is only a fraction of a training year, but the sample programs should give you insight into the process of designing programs. The final sample program demonstrates how to improve lateral movement and change of direction skills for a young tennis player.

EXERCISE VARIABLES

Any training program should begin with a period of preparation and move into time frames, or cycles, with specific goals. An example would be a six week cycle that begins with a pretest and has the goal of increased distance in the standing triple jump. The cycle would end with a posttest to see if the goal was achieved. An effective program accomplishes specific goals through the manipulation of four variables: intensity, volume, frequency, and recovery.

INTENSITY

Intensity is the effort involved in performing a given task. In weightlifting, intensity is controlled by the amount of weight lifted. In plyometrics, intensity is controlled by the type of exercise performed. Plyometrics ranges from simple tasks to highly complex and stressful exercises. Starting out with skipping is much less stressful than alternate bounding. Double leg hops are less intense than single leg bounds.

The intensity of plyometric exercises can be increased by adding light weights in certain cases, by raising the platform height for depth jumps, or simply by aiming at covering a greater distance in longitudinal jumps. Other writers have rated the intensity of various plyometric exercises from low to very intense (Stone and O'Bryant, 1987). The exercises in this book are rated low to high. Any attempt to classify exercises by intensity is imperfect at best, but the guidelines provided here should help you in your program design. Figure 3.1 depicts the scale of intensity for jump training exercises.

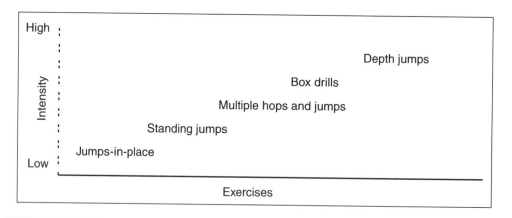

Figure 3.1   Intensity scale for jump training exercises.

VOLUME

Volume is the total work performed in a single workout session or cycle. In the case of plyometric training, volume is often measured by counting foot contacts. For example, an activity like the standing triple jump, comprised of three parts, counts as three foot contacts. Foot contacts provide a means of prescribing and monitoring exercise volume.

The recommended volume of specific jumps in any one session will vary with intensity and progression goals. Table 3.1 shows sample exercise volumes for beginning, intermediate, and advanced workouts. A beginner in a single workout in an off-season cycle could do 60 to 100 foot contacts of low-intensity exercises. The intermediate exerciser might be able to do 100 to 150 foot contacts of low-intensity exercises and another 100 of moderate-intensity exercises in the same cycle. Advanced exercisers might be capable of 150 to 250 foot contacts of low- to moderate-intensity exercises in this cycle.

The volume of bounding (exaggerated running) activities is best measured by distance. In the early phases of conditioning, a reasonable distance is

TABLE 3.1   NUMBER OF FOOT CONTACTS BY SEASON FOR JUMP TRAINING

	Level			
	Beginning	**Intermediate**	**Advanced**	**Intensity**
Off-season	60-100	100-150	120-200	Low-Mod
Preseason	100-250	150-300	150-450	Mod-High
In-season	Depends on sport			Moderate
Championship season	Recovery only			Mod-High

30 meters per repetition. As the season progresses and the abilities of athletes improve, the distance may be progressively increased to 100 meters per repetition.

Low-intensity exercises used during warm-ups are generally not included in the number of foot contacts when computing volume. Thus warm-ups should stay low in intensity and progressive in nature so they do not overextend the athlete.

FREQUENCY

Frequency is the number of times an exercise is performed (repetitions) as well as the number of times exercise sessions take place during a training cycle.

Research on frequency in plyometrics is obscure. There seems to be no conclusive evidence that one frequency pattern is the means of increasing performance. Practical experience and some European writings have led me to believe that 48 to 72 hours of rest is necessary for full recovery before the next exercise stimulus, although the intensity of the exercises has to be considered. Skipping as a plyometric exercise is not as stressful as bounding and will not require the same amount of recovery time. Beginners should have at least 48 hours of recovery between plyometric sessions. If the athlete does not get enough recovery, muscle fatigue results in the athlete's being unable to respond to the exercise stimuli (ground contact, distance, height) with maximal, quality efforts. The overall result is less efficient training for athletic development.

There are varied methods for establishing frequency in plyometric training. Some coaches prefer to use a Monday and Thursday schedule during the preparation cycle (see table 3.2). Using the principle of 48 to 72 hours of

TABLE 3.2   SAMPLES OF FREQUENCY OF OFF-SEASON OR PRESEASON PLYOMETRIC TRAINING

	Program 1	Program 2	Program 3
Monday	Weight training	Plyometrics (lower extremities)	Plyometrics (lower extremities)
Tuesday	Plyometrics (lower extremities)	Weight training	Plyometrics (upper extremities—medicine ball)
Wednesday	Weight training	Plyometrics (upper extremities—medicine ball)	Running program
Thursday	Plyometrics (lower extremities)	Weight training	Plyometrics (lower extremities)
Friday	Weight training	Plyometrics (lower extremities)	Rest

recovery for lower extremity training, one can easily see the many program variations that can be developed. Running programs can also be integrated into the training cycle along with or replacing weight training on certain days, although it is recommended that weight training be a priority in developing and maintaining the strength base necessary to carry out a successful plyometric training program.

Because of the stressful nature of plyometrics and the emphasis on quality of work, plyometric exercises should be performed before any other exercise programs. They can be integrated into weight training (this combination, called complex training, is described later in this chapter) at a later cycle in the training year if desired, or they might comprise the entire workout. This is quite conceivable, in fact, if the athlete is involved in track and field, where the plyometric training might be very specific to the event or to skill development.

RECOVERY

Recovery is a key variable in determining whether plyometrics will succeed in developing power or muscular endurance. For power training, longer recovery periods (45 to 60 seconds) between sets or groupings of multiple events, such as a set of 10 rim jumps, allow maximum recovery between efforts. A work to rest ratio of 1:5 to 1:10 is required to assure proper execution and intensity of the exercise. Thus, if a single set of exercises takes 10 seconds to complete, 50 to 100 seconds of recovery should be allowed. Remember, plyometric training is an anaerobic activity. Shorter recovery periods (10 to 15 seconds) between sets do not allow for maximum recovery of muscular endurance.

Less than two seconds of recovery time in a 12 to 20 minute workout makes it aerobic. Exercise for both strength and endurance is usually achieved through circuit training, where the athlete continues from one exercise to another without stopping between sets.

The preparation (off-season) cycle for a plyometric program should involve general gross motor exercises, such as skipping for coordination or simple jumping, without specific skill training like change of direction. As the pre-season cycle approaches, exercises should become more specific to the sport.

If the sport itself is specific to plyometric training, as in long, high, and triple jumping, plyometrics can be carried through the in-season cycle. However, for sports dominated by vertical jumping, like basketball and volleyball, it may be advisable to reduce the amount of plyometric training to a level consistent with the development of the athlete. For example, a professional basketball team that plays a schedule of three or more games a week with constant travel may find it impossible to train plyometrically during the season. On the other hand, the men's national volleyball team conducts plyometric training of up to 400 jumps while training during the season because they play a limited match schedule. Common sense must play a role in determining whether the athlete should continue plyometrics in season.

USING PLYOMETRICS WITH OTHER TRAINING

Jump training and upper body plyometrics are relevant to many sports. Gymnastics, jumping events in track and field, diving, and volleyball are all arenas where success depends on the athlete's ability to explode from the standing surface and generate vertical velocity, linear velocity, or both to achieve the desired result.

But plyometrics is not a panacea in athletic conditioning. It does not exist in a vacuum, nor should it be thought of as a singular form of training. Instead, plyometrics is the icing on the cake, to be used by athletes who have prepared their tendons and muscles through resistance training for the tremendous impact forces imposed in high-intensity plyometrics.

Anaerobic conditioning, in the form of sprint or interval training, is essential to developing the stride patterns required in proper plyometric bounding. The explosive reactions of sprinting or of movement drills that require changes of direction can be performed as interval training (repeated efforts with measured recovery periods).

Done together, resistance training and anaerobic training help prepare the athlete's body for plyometrics. In turn, plyometrics enhances the athlete's ability to perform in resistance exercise and anaerobic activity—a true partnership in athletic training.

RESISTANCE TRAINING

Resistance training is the ideal counterpart of plyometric training for it helps prepare the muscles for the rapid impact loading of plyometric exercises. In resistance training one works to develop the eccentric phase of muscle contraction by first lowering the body or weight and then overcoming the weight using a concentric contraction.

Open-chain resistance training (using machines that isolate a single joint) is useful for developing strength in specific muscle groups. However, the user of plyometrics also needs to perform closed-chain exercises that involve multi-joint activities such as free weight exercises (using barbells, dumbbells, and a medicine ball). These exercises, which are generally performed with the feet fixed to the ground as in squatting, are more functional for athletes, allowing them to assume positions specific to their sports when they exercise. Closed-chain exercises have proven themselves to have much higher carryover value than isolated joint exercises in developing athletic ability.

Plyometric training can be successfully integrated with resistance training by imposing a speed-strength task immediately on muscles that have been subjected to pure strength movements like those in weightlifting (see the discussion of complex training on page 65).

The more intense plyometric exercises become, the more crucial the need for strength. As mentioned earlier, some of the early European literature spoke of the need to squat 2.5 times body weight before undergoing a training program. There is no doubt that those authors had a high-intensity program in mind, but a strength requirement is part and parcel of plyometric training at all levels.

Parameters that are used to determine if an athlete is strong enough to begin a plyometric program may center more on functional strength (including power) testing than the traditional one-repetition maximum (1 RM) squat that measures pure strength. One such test has been used by a number of practitioners in plyometric training programs. As a test of power more than strength, it may have more direct applicability.

Weight equal to 60 percent of the athlete's body weight is placed on a squat bar, and the athlete is asked to perform five repetitions in five seconds, tested against a stopwatch. If the athlete cannot do so, emphasis should be given to a resistance training program and the intensity of the plyometric training program should remain low to moderate.

Poor strength in the lower extremities results in loss of stability when landing, and high-impact forces are excessively absorbed by the soft tissues of the body. Early fatigue also becomes a problem without adequate leg strength. Together, these will result in the deterioration of performance during exercise and an increased chance for injury (as in any overuse situation).

ANAEROBIC, SPRINT, AND INTERVAL TRAINING

Plyometrics trains two anaerobic energy systems, the creatine phosphate and the lactic acid cycles. The creatine phosphate system depends on energy stores that already exist in the muscles. Plyometric exercises that last a mere

4 to 15 seconds deplete the energy stores. When designing a program to train the creatine phosphate system, a considerable amount of rest or recovery should be allotted between exercises; the emphasis is on quality of work, not quantity. The lactic acid threshold is reached when the muscles' energy stores have been exhausted by the creatine phosphate system. Exercise that proceeds past the point of using the energy stores taxes the lactic acid threshold. Exercise bouts at near-maximal effort that last around 30 to 90 seconds are appropriate for training that system.

In general, jumps-in-place, standing jumps, and depth jumps are short-duration activities used to train the creatine phosphate system. Multiple jumps, box drills, and particularly bounding can qualify as exercises for training the lactic acid threshold.

It is beneficial to train the creatine phosphate system in athletes involved in sports that require quick bursts of power with long recovery periods between performances, such as the long jump or triple jump. Training the lactic acid threshold is helpful for athletes in sports like football or volleyball where activity is fairly prolonged and rest periods are more infrequent.

Sprint and interval training are running programs that require the athlete to perform quality efforts in training for a certain amount of time (usually around 30 to 90 seconds) with prescribed recovery periods. This type of training is closely related to plyometric training of the lactic acid threshold but uses sprints instead of multiple jumps, box drills, or bounding exercises.

CIRCUIT TRAINING

One of the many benefits of plyometric training is that it can be organized into circuits. By moving from station to station (see figure 3.2), the athlete can do a variety of exercises that stress either the vertical or linear components of various movement patterns, or both.

By using circuits, athletes can perform activities of even greater duration than with anaerobic, sprint, and interval training. This may move the level of cardiovascular stress toward improvement in aerobic conditioning, resulting in increased stamina. The cumulative effect of circuit training is considerable, so the recovery period should be at least two days.

DESIGNING A BASIC PROGRAM

A basic plyometric program might be intended for the novice or the young athlete. It should follow the rules of safety and the considerations set forth in chapter 2. If the program is intended for the more advanced athlete, the same rules apply, but the exercises become more complex and more intense. The following considerations affect the design of training programs at any level.

TESTING AND ASSESSMENT

I cannot, of course, attempt to detail the hundreds of physical tests that exist in sport. But it is important to know that testing (data collection) and

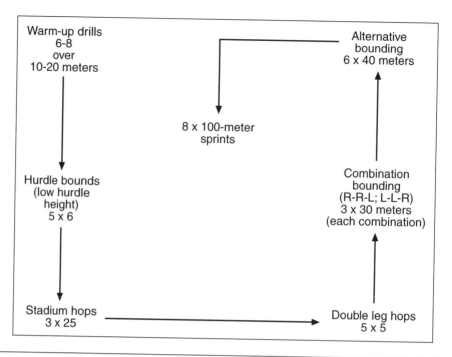

Figure 3.2　Sample circuit.

assessment (comparing the gathered data to establish performance standards) of an athlete before and after training periods, or cycles, is vital to both measuring improvement and providing direction and motivation. Goal setting should be a way of life for athletes and coaches. Most athletes respond positively to definable goals and reasonable standards.

Standard tests of physical fitness, such as the 300-yard shuttle, the standing vertical jump, and the standing long jump, are good for gathering baseline data. These or similar test scores should be recorded for future reference. More advanced athletes can be tested on skills such as the standing triple jump or the single leg hop over 25 meters.

Plyometric training should be a means of improving self-image and self-realization. Athletes should be concerned with competing against themselves and should be encouraged to do as well as they can in training as well as testing. Testing should be done both before and after training modules to let athletes rate themselves against their own accomplishments as well as against established norms.

For athletes in individual events, such as track and field or swimming, the ultimate posttest is the competition itself—even more so during the championship season. It is there that the time spent in preparation, planning, and performance can culminate in that moment of synthesis known as peaking.

MOVEMENT SKILLS

Teach beginners the concepts behind plyometric activities, including the importance of eccentric versus concentric strength. Stress the importance of the stretch-shortening cycle (the countermovement of the legs) in the ability to start quickly.

Feet should be nearly flat in all landings. The ball of the foot may touch first, but the rest of the foot should also make contact. Landing should be reversed quickly; the object is to spend minimal time on the ground.

For the arms to help develop force into the ground to "compress the spring," elbows must be brought behind the midline of the body so the arms can be brought rapidly forward and up as the concentric contraction occurs for liftoff. This movement is the double arm swing.

Initial activities should be of lower intensity (see chapter 4 for examples) and preparatory. The coach must be aware of the progression needed in both intensity and skill requirement.

TIME

Actual exercise time in a beginning plyometric program should not exceed 20 to 30 minutes. An additional 10 to 15 minutes each should be devoted to a warm-up and a cool-down that emphasize stretching and low-intensity movement activities. Warm-ups can start with passive stretching and walking and progress to skipping, light jogging, and side-to-side movements, using big arm swings to warm up the shoulders. Cool-downs should focus on low-stress activities such as light jogging, stretching, and walking. Advanced athletes may do longer workouts to perform longer drills, requiring greater recovery.

PLYOMETRIC ACTIVITY

The actual number of jumps to be implemented in any program depends on many variables. Remember that this is a sample program, and your particular situation might call for variation. Refer to the information on intensity, frequency, volume, and recovery earlier in this chapter. The key guiding concepts are prudence and simplicity.

Some variables concern whether an athlete is involved in complementary resistance or weight training. An athlete without prior experience generally should not perform plyometric and resistance training on the same day. An experienced athlete who wishes to combine plyometrics and resistance training should do plyometrics first to allow for maximal response from muscles not fatigued by prior exertions. Plyometrics and weight training can also be effectively combined by advanced or elite athletes in complex training (page 65).

Another concern regarding plyometric training is the timing of the athletic season. In the off-season or preseason, training should progress toward more intense exercises. To supplement in-season training, conditioning levels should be maintained using exercises of low to moderate intensity.

Prudence in prescribing and performing plyometric exercise has to do with when and how much training is done. A hard, skill-oriented sport practice should not be followed by a high-volume, high-intensity plyometric workout. More will be accomplished by using warm-up and low-intensity plyometric work to allow for recovery. Even better would be devoting a single training day to plyometrics to provide variety and allow physiological and mental recovery from skill practice.

LENGTH OF CYCLE

The length of time spent in any single training cycle depends on the days per week available before the start of the season. With beginning athletes, the emphasis should be on skill development, not on progression to higher intensity exercises. Twelve to 18 weeks of a basic plyometric program is advised to ensure that athletes can properly execute the mechanics of plyometric activities before they attempt higher volumes and intensities of exercise. This is compatible with the off-season and preseason cycles of training format discussed under the topic of volume in this chapter.

SAFETY

Probably the most important safety consideration to remember is that more is not necessarily better. If a workout has been accomplished with apparent ease, go back to the drawing board for future workouts. Don't impulsively add more exercises that day just because there's no visible fatigue. Remember that quality, not quantity, is the goal in plyometric training.

The abilities and body composition of the individual also affect the safety of training. Large, heavy athletes should not perform single leg activities until they have fully adjusted to the stress of plyometric training. It would not be unusual for such athletes to do double leg jumps for an entire season before developing the necessary strength for more complex activities (standing triple jumps, single leg hops, etc.). This same conservative philosophy applies to young athletes without strength or jump training experience.

Staying physically healthy is a must we take for granted, but it requires planning. Coaches must make sure that their plyometric training programs do not increase an athlete's chances of injury. Often injuries occur when muscles are tired—at the end of practice or when the coach asks for "just one more." Fatigue takes away from the sharpness of senses, and the athlete is probably just going through the motions of the exercise. Sprained ankles and twisted knees are among the common trauma associated with a lack of control due to excessive fatigue. This is the time when prudence is particularly important.

A final safety consideration concerns the overload principle. In extending this principle to plyometrics, coaches ask, "Should athletes use weights when they jump?" It is not advisable for beginning athletes to use any weighted vests, belts, or bands. Although the earlier European writings describe the use of added weight (up to 10 percent of body weight), this was with elite athletes with years of experience in training and competition. And even these athletes were not continuously subjected to this regimen. Adding weight should be done with caution, only after a long preparation period, and no more than once a week for an eight week cycle.

THE SPORT-SPECIFIC PROGRAM

Creating a sport-specific program requires understanding the mechanics of the sport by doing a needs analysis, breaking down skill patterns into their most elementary parts. For example, a volleyball spike depends largely on being able to make a short approach, convert horizontal movement into vertical lift, and perform a swinging motion at the top of the jump. Plyometric work, then, should focus on developing the vertical component of jumping. But a football running back, by contrast, must develop great horizontal acceleration from a static start and needs tremendous lateral hip strength for rapid changes of direction. In plyometric training, 80 percent of total foot contacts should apply to activities that closely resemble the skills necessary for success in the sport; the remaining 20 percent can apply to general conditioning.

As an athlete develops, so will the ability to use plyometrics. A long or triple jumper, for example, often uses plyometric training for both conditioning and skill development because the event is close to the exercise itself. It is not unusual for a college triple or long jumper to start out bounding 300 total meters per exercise session and by midseason do 1,500 total meters of bounding in a single workout.

In other sports, such as basketball, volleyball, tennis, and football, various jump drills can be integrated with skill patterns to approximate what happens on the court or field. Table 3.3 shows what skills are developed by which jump.

TABLE 3.3　SKILLS BUILT BY PLYOMETRIC EXERCISE

Skill	Jumps-in-place	Standing jumps	Multiple jumps	Box drills	Bounding	Depth jumps
Start speed	✓	✓	✓			✓
Acceleration			✓	✓	✓	
Change of direction		✓	✓	✓		✓
Vertical jump	✓	✓	✓	✓		✓
Horizontal jump		✓	✓	✓	✓	

THE SYNCHRONIZED SWIMMER

The goal is to develop a program which will increase her power in the upper extremities and help develop the stabilizing muscles of the shoulder.

STEP 1: CONSIDER THE ATHLETE

Kristina is a 17-year-old synchronized swimmer. She is ranked high on the age-group and national levels. She has no experience in resistance training and has chronic shoulder pain due to a condition known as multidirectional instability in both shoulders.

STEP 2: ASSESS AND TEST THE ATHLETE

1. *Push-ups.* Assume a push-up position with the hands resting on the ground directly under the shoulders and the body in straight alignment, off the ground from the toes. Count how many the athlete can perform in 30 seconds.

2. *Overhead medicine ball throw for distance.* Assume a standing position one step behind a tape line with the ball held behind the head with both hands. Take one step forward, and throw the ball overhead as far as you can. Do not step over or on the tape line. Measure the distance from the tape line to the spot where the ball hits the ground.

3. *Medicine ball chest pass.* Assume a seated position on a ground surface with the back against the wall and the legs straight out. The ball is held at midchest with both hands. On command, attempt to pass the ball as far as you can. The distance thrown is measured from your heels to the spot where the ball hits the ground.

4. *Sit-ups for time.* This test is a measure of trunk power. The athlete is on her back, legs bent, feet resting flat on the floor and secured by the tester. Hands are interlocked and placed on the area behind the neck. The athlete is asked to perform as many successful sit-ups (defined as a trunk movement resulting in the elbows touching the thighs) as possible within a 30-second time frame.

These tests are an indication of the strength and power that Kristina has in the upper extremities and trunk. As expected, her push-up score is a very low 8, with the acceptable score as used by the United States Synchronized Swimming Association being 30. Her medicine ball overhead throw is 12'8", with the average score of other synchronized swimmers in her age bracket being 23'. Her chest pass score is 8'9", with an average score of other similar athletes being 18'6". Finally, her sit-up score was 22, placing her two standard deviations below the mean score for elite junior synchronized swimmers.

The overall assessment is that we have an athlete deficient in terms of strength and power in the upper extremities. Her multidirectional instability obviously affects her performance on these tests.

We need to design a program that will strengthen the shoulders as well as teach the athlete how to exert force rapidly. The metabolism utilized by synchronized swimmers is long-term anaerobic; therefore, endurance and stamina are as important to success as raw strength and power. Another important consideration is the amount of practice time devoted to this sport and her current ability to function in the water.

STEP 3: CONSIDER THE TIME FRAME OR CYCLE

Kristina is at the beginning of her season, which starts just after the Labor Day holiday in September. Her season is pointed entirely toward success in the national competition held in mid-April. She has the ability to work out three times a week until February, when her pool time becomes so extensive that two times per week maximum will be available for dry land training.

Given her current physical status and test scores, the preparation cycle is crucial to her success this year.

STEP 4: SELECT THE TIME IN THE TRAINING YEAR

With the above information and the knowledge that preparation is the key to Kristina having a good chance to perform well throughout the season, we would be well advised to plan carefully and focus on the first six week cycle.

STEP 5: DESIGN THE PROGRAM

WEEKS 1-4

PREPARATION

Since the test scores indicate large deficiencies in upper extremity strength and power we will develop a program that focuses on overcoming just that.

PROGRESSION

Using moderate- to high-volume, low-intensity resistance training we will develop strategic areas of the shoulder to help overcome the instability problem. The medicine ball will be a key tool to our implementing this program.

EXERCISE FREQUENCY

Three days a week (Tuesday, Thursday, and Saturday) at the pool.

LIMITATIONS

Little to no equipment. Basically a gymnastics mat large enough to hold 10 athletes and medicine balls of weights that vary in 2-pound increments from 6 to 12 pounds.

EXERCISES

- 3×8 push-ups that require the athlete to touch her chest to the ball in the down position. The purpose of the ball is to provide a target that limits the excursion of the exercises, therefore assuring completion of them.
- 3×5 offset push-ups that require the athlete to place one hand on the ball and perform the push-up movement. The purpose of placing one hand on the ball is that it forces the athlete to stabilize the shoulder with the hand on the ball to a greater degree, since the ball is a somewhat unstable surface.
- 3×5 close grip push-ups performed with both hands on the ball. This sets up a difficult angle for the arms to perform the push-ups while adding the element of instability to increase forced stability.
- 1×30 pull-over passes
- 1×30 underhand throws
- 2×20 power drops
- 2×20 side tosses
- 1×15 overhead throws

WEEKS 4-8

PROGRESSION

Increase the number of repetitions during the push-up activities by two to three each week. By weeks 4-8 add the following:

- 1×30 seconds of the walkabout. This is performed by assuming the push-up position with one hand on the ball and one hand on the ground. The athlete transfers the on-the-ground hand to rest next to the one on the ball. The hand on the ball then moves to the ground on that side. The alternating of the hands results in the athlete moving across the top of the ball in a "walking" sort of way.

By week 8 the following may also be a possibility:

- 1×10 medicine ball depth jumps, performed by starting in the push-up position with both hands on the ball. The athlete "drops" from being on the ball to a position where both hands are on the ground with the elbows slightly flexed. By rapidly extending the arms and generating shoulder push the athlete "jumps" from the ground to the starting position.

The latter exercises call into play the rather quick contraction of the stabilizing muscles around the shoulder. This theory goes back to what the East Europeans called "shock" training, in which "shocking" the stabilizers of the shoulder trains them to contract rapidly and function more effectively.

Preparation needs for this type of athlete under these conditions is not a rarity. Indeed, many coaches, athletes, and strength coaches are faced with similar situations. When there is little in the way of resources, equipment, and time, the athlete will suffer unless the coaches can be creative.

THE BASEBALL PLAYER

Bat speed and trunk power are a priority.

STEP 1: CONSIDER THE ATHLETE

Jerry is a 23-year-old professional baseball player. He has been on the road for several months after the baseball season. Vacation, business interests, etc., have consumed much of his time. He has now decided to put serious time into getting ready for spring ball. He has been lifting on his own and has a fair level of strength development. As a first baseman, he is not expected to possess great sprint speed. He is, however, expected to produce hits and runs.

STEP 2: ASSESS AND TEST THE ATHLETE

In this case we are presented with a physically gifted athlete who has been through a long season of playing competitive baseball games. The most important thing is that the individual has asked to be subjected to a program which will be of six weeks duration, the goal of which is to prepare him for camp. The ultimate assessment is his performance in that baseball camp.

STEP 3: CONSIDER THE TIME FRAME OR CYCLE

Jerry has six weeks to get ready. We must develop a program that will maximize the benefits without resulting in overtraining or injury.

STEP 4: SELECT THE TIME IN THE TRAINING YEAR

The time is definitely preseason and is to coincide with the beginning of spring training.

STEP 5: DESIGN THE PROGRAM

WEEKS 1-3

PREPARATION

This program will use several variations due to the short time interval available for training. Several variations of complex training will be used, with special emphasis on developing core or trunk strength. Given his reputation as a hitter, the program must emphasize those areas that will get the majority of stress once he sets foot in camp.

PROGRESSION

This program will be divided into two cycles of three weeks each. The first three weeks will include resistance training exercises and plyometric drills to emphasize fundamental movements. Many of the exercises are grouped via their relationship to each other by muscle groups or total body function. The second cycle will emphasize sport-specific drills as well as plyometric activities to increase speed of movement. The medicine ball drills for core strength are changed every two weeks.

DAY 1

- 3×8 front squats followed by 3×8 push presses
- 3×10 inclined hammer curls followed by 3×10 bicep pull-downs on the lat machine
- 3×8 chest presses on the machine followed by 3×8 seated rows

CORE STRENGTH: MEDICINE BALL WORK (FIRST TWO WEEKS)

Trunk rotation (10 reps each direction)

Alternating toe touch (10 reps each side)

Hip rolls (10 reps each direction)

Offset push-ups (10 each side)

Repeat this circuit twice.

Seated toe touch (15 reps)

Sit-up toss (15 reps)

Bridge with both feet on medicine ball (15 reps)

Superman arch (15 reps)

Repeat this circuit twice.

DAY 2

- 3×10 back squats, each set to be followed by 1×10 jumps to the box (24-inch)
- 3×6 behind the neck presses, each set to be followed by 1×10 overhead medicine ball throws at maximum effort
- 3×10 lat pull-downs, each set to be followed by 1×10 medicine ball pull-over tosses
- 3×8 torso rotations, each set to be followed by 1×12 reps of side throws and 12 over-and-back throws (each side)

Same medicine ball work as Day 1.

DAY 3

- 3×10 step-ups, each set to be followed by 1×10 side lunges (each side), followed by 1 set of walking L lunges over a distance of 20 yards
- 3×10 hang cleans, each set to be followed by a set of six hurdle jumps (30-inch)
- 3×3 lateral hurdle hops (18-inch) to be repeated five times
- 5 sets of hexagon drills (each drill includes three trips around the hexagon)
- 4×6 hamstring curls, 3×30 yards of heel kick running drills to follow these sets

Same medicine ball work as Day 1.

PROGRESSION

Core Strength program should change after the first two weeks and include the following for the next two weeks:

Alternating toe touch (15 reps each side)

Hip rolls (15 reps each direction)

Sit-up passes (25 reps)

Power drops (25 reps)

Repeat this circuit three times.

Russian twist (15 reps)

Single leg bridging (15 reps each leg)

Standing side throws (20 reps each side)

Hands on the ball push-ups (15 reps)

Repeat this circuit three times.

WEEKS 4-6

The final three weeks of training will include more sport-specific and speed-of-movement drills, along with functional resistance training.

DAY 1

- 3×12 on the Multi-Hip Machine working hip flexion, extension, abduction, and adduction
- 1×10 lateral change of direction drills for maximal effort
- The player practices hitting a baseball that has been soft tossed into a net with the Frappier resistance cords attached to the hips and arms. The cords are removed immediately after he hits 40 to 50 balls, and he hits freely for another 40 to 50 balls. This represents a form of contrast training to improve trunk rotation speed.

MEDICINE BALL DRILLS FOR CORE STRENGTH

Use the above program for weeks 3 and 4, then progress to the following program for weeks 5 and 6.

DAY 2

- 1×10 four-way lunges (front, 45 degree, side, and crossover)
- Frappier footwork drills (approximately 30 minutes of various routines)
- Medicine ball drills for core strength

Interval speed running workout on treadmill (approximately one hour in length)

DAY 3

Repeat Day 1.

The final two weeks of Core Strength exercises utilizing the medicine ball are as follows:

Chinnies (45-60 seconds)

Superman toss (15 reps)

Diagonal toss (15 reps each side)

Walkabouts (30 seconds)

Repeat this circuit twice.

Trunk rotation (15 reps each side)

Hip rolls (15 reps each direction)

Russian twists (15 reps each side)

Over-and-back toss (20 reps)

Standing diagonal throw (12 reps)

Repeat this circuit three times.

The Soccer Player

Before leaving for an NCAA Division I college program, Brooke wants to develop skills that will impress her college coaches.

Step 1: Consider the Athlete

Brooke is a 17-year-old female soccer player who is preparing to leave for an NCAA Division I college program. She has 12 weeks to prepare for her introduction to the collegiate level of competition. She is still involved in summer club playing, yet feels she needs to do extra work if she is going to make the desired impression on the college coaches.

Step 2: Assess and Test the Athlete

Brooke is 5'9" tall and weighs 137 pounds. She has lifted on an irregular basis in the past. Her background also includes experience in performing basic plyometric training.

1. *Standing jump-and-reach.* Brooke has a standing jump-and-reach score of 15 inches.

2. *Maximum squat.* Brooke is able to do a 95-pound maximum squat for three reps.

3. *Bench press.* Testing for a 1 RM score in the bench press gives us some indication of her basic upper body strength. Her maximum effort was 55 pounds.

4. *T test.* This test is performed on a T that is 10 yards across the top and has a 10-yard stem. The athlete starts at the base of the stem, running forward, then shuffling to the right or left along the top of the T until both ends are touched. The athlete then returns to the middle and backpedals along the stem to the original start position. Her score is 10.2 seconds. The average score for the collegiate female soccer player is 10.8 seconds.

5. *Sit-up test for 30 seconds.* Since throw-ins in soccer are a function of core strength, this test is an indicator of the need for trunk strengthening. Brooke completes 20 sit-ups in 30 seconds.

All of the scores indicate that we are dealing with a young athlete who has been able to compete at the high school level because of her soccer skills and speed. Being quick and skillful would make her a candidate for recruiting; however, survival at the next level is going to require strength, power, and physical stamina.

Step 3: Consider the Time Frame or Cycle

Brooke has three months in which to develop her overall physical strength and endurance. Her continued desire to play soccer during this time might become a conflict. However, she is willing to split her workout days, insuring she will spend three days per week training with the weights and plyometrics.

Step 4: Select the Time in the Training Year

Brooke has to devote the summer months after graduation from high school until she reports to her university for school and practice. Each cycle can fit well into a four week block.

STEP 5: DESIGN THE PROGRAM

The basic needs of this athlete are general strength and power development with specific emphasis on vertical jump, core strength, and both upper and lower body strength development.

WEEKS 1-4

DAY 1

- 3×12 hamstring curls
- 3×10 leg presses
- 3×12 lat pull-downs
- 3×10 shoulder presses
- 3×10 bench presses
- 2×12 back hyperextensions
- 3×8 torso rotations

CORE STRENGTH: MEDICINE BALL WORK

Sit-up straight arm (15 reps)

Pull-over pass (15 reps)

Alternate toe touch (10 reps each side)

Side toss (15 reps each side)

Backward toss (15 reps)

Front toss (10 reps)

Heel toss (10 reps)

DAY 2

- 2×10 split squats (each side)
- 2×10 dumbbell presses
- 3×6 front squat to shoulder presses
- Frappier footwork patterns, up to 2:30 minutes total time
- Four square pattern (any combination of squares may be used; see page 72)
- 5×6 front cone hops
- 3×6 lateral cone hops (each direction)
- 1×30 seconds single leg push-offs (12-inch box)
- 1×30 seconds side-to-side (12-inch box)

DAY 3

Repeat Day 1.

WEEKS 5-8

PROGRESSION

The goal is to advance Brooke into more dynamic activities that challenge her, yet provide continuous strength gains.

DAY 1

- 3 × 8 front squats
- 2 × 10 lunges (both legs)
- 3 × 8 push presses
- 3 × 8 seated rows
- 3 × 8 incline bench presses
- 3 × 10 dumbbell pull-over

CORE STRENGTH: MEDICINE BALL WORK

Sit-up pass (15 reps)

Pull-over pass (15 reps)

Hip crunches (15 reps)

Russian twists (10 reps)

Side toss (15 reps each side)

Hip rolls (10 reps each side)

Backward throw (10 reps)

Front toss (15 reps)

Heel toss (10 reps)

Repeat this circuit twice.

DAY 2

- 3 × 10 lat pull-downs, each set followed by 10 overhead throws
- 3 × 8 bench presses, each set followed by 12 power drops
- 3 × 10 heel tosses with medicine ball
- 3 sets of hexagon drills
- 3 × 3 lateral hurdle (12-inch) hops (hop down, back, and down without stopping)
- 3 × 10 depth jumps (18-inch box)
- 3 × 30 seconds box drills (12-inch box)
- 3 × 20 yards skipping
- 3 × 20 yards power skipping
- 3 × 20 yards single leg hops

DAY 3

Repeat Day 1.

WEEKS 9-12

COMPETITION

Power development becomes the main focus of this final cycle. Lifting loads should be reduced to 30 to 60 percent 1 RM so that the bar can be moved rapidly. This allows for maximal power development through the full range of motion. Plyometric drills should be related, as often as possible, to the specific movements in soccer.

DAY 1

- 4 sets of 5-5-5 squats
- 4×5 push presses
- 4×5 high pulls (clean grip)
- 4×5 single leg squats (each leg)
- 3×8 depth jumps (18-inch box)
- 2×8 180-degree turn depth jumps (18-inch box) (both directions)
- 5×6 hurdle hops (24-inch)
- 1×60 seconds box drill

DAY 2

CORE STRENGTH: MEDICINE BALL WORK

Sit-up pass (25 reps)

Pull-over pass (25 reps)

Diagonal toss (20 reps each side)

Trunk rotation (12 reps each side)

Hip rolls (20 reps each side)

Repeat this circuit twice.

Overhead throw (15 reps for maximum distance)

Backward throw (10 reps for maximum distance)

Front toss (20 reps)

Heel toss (15 reps)

Repeat this circuit three times.

PLYOMETRIC DRILLS

- 3×30 yards skipping

- 3×30 yards power skipping
- 3×30 yards single arm alternate bounding
- 5×5 double leg hops

DAY 3

Repeat Day 1.

The intensity of this third cycle is very high and will depend on Brooke's ability to gain strength and demonstrate an adequate level of adaptation to the plyometric training. If she fails to do so, the exercise intensity will be lowered and lower-level plyometrics substituted.

SAMPLE PROGRAMS FOR INCREASING VERTICAL AND LINEAR JUMPS

The following are two specific sample programs, one that develops vertical jumping and one that develops linear jumping. The sample programs are based on the specific needs of the hypothetical athletes described. For this reason they are not to be applied universally, but you can adapt the principles to design programs specific to your needs.

VERTICAL JUMP

There is a five-step procedure that can be followed to improve vertical jump. For the sake of brevity, this sample program covers only four weeks of a training cycle.

STEP 1: CONSIDER THE ATHLETE

James is a 16-year-old basketball player with one year of varsity experience. He has had two years of resistance training in the high school football coach's weightlifting class. He has sprained an ankle in the past, but he is healthy at this time.

STEP 2: ASSESS AND TEST THE ATHLETE

For developing vertical jump, measure the following abilities:

1. *Standing jump-and-reach.* Standing on both feet, James reaches as high as he can on a wall; mark that height. Then James jumps off both feet and reaches as high on the wall as he can; again mark the height. Record the difference between the two marks.

2. *Jump from box.* James does a depth jump from an 18-inch box. After he lands, he jumps up and reaches as high on the wall as he can; record the height of the touch.

3. *Three-step vertical jump.* James takes three steps and on the final step (which should be with his preferred foot) jumps up and reaches as high on the wall as he can; mark the height of the jump.

4. *One-repetition maximum parallel squat.* James determines the maximum amount of weight he can lift one time doing a back squat. To do the squat, James stands with his back to a barbell that is resting on a rack at shoulder height, lifts the barbell to rest on his shoulders, bends at the hips and knees until his thighs are parallel to the floor, and returns to the starting position.

5. *Five-repetition/five-second parallel squat at 60 percent body weight.* James performs five squats with a barbell, weighted equal to 60 percent of his body weight. He attempts to do the squats within five seconds.

The test results dictate the type and direction of the program. For James, Tests 4 and 5 indicate adequate strength because his 1 RM squat was 1.5 times his body weight, and he could squat five times in five seconds with 60 percent of his body weight. If these scores had been below standard (he could squat only 75 percent of his body weight and took 7.5 seconds to complete five squats at 60 percent of his body weight), it would indicate that resistance work is still a major requirement of training or even a prerequisite to undergoing high-intensity plyometrics. Strength work alone might increase vertical jump if James were deficient.

Tests 1, 2, and 3 show James's present vertical jumping ability and give data against which to measure his progress at the end of the program. James reached 21 inches in the standing jump-and-reach, 18 inches in the jump from box, and 20 inches in the three-step vertical jump (indicating that he isn't any better off one foot than two).

STEP 3: CONSIDER THE TIME FRAME OR CYCLE

James's program will be for four weeks. The program has been condensed from a normal periodized training year to demonstrate the preparation, progression, and performance variables involved in program design. At the end of this cycle, James is retested to check for progress.

STEP 4: SELECT THE TIME IN THE TRAINING YEAR

James will follow his program during the month of September, before the onset of the season and at the time when most high school athletes in winter sports begin to make an effort to get in shape.

STEP 5: DESIGN THE PROGRAM

Plan each of the four weeks according to three variables:

1. Preparation
2. Progression
3. Performance

WEEK 1

PREPARATION

Use high-volume, low-intensity resistance training and low-intensity plyometrics to allow the body's soft tissues to accommodate to the stress of jumping and the impact of landing.

PROGRESSION

Include enough variety to challenge the athlete to learn new skills.

PERFORMANCE

Concentrate on proper landing techniques and the use of the arms in performing low-intensity exercises. Make sure the concept of the amortization phase is understood.

WORKOUT SCHEDULE

Remember, this is a hypothetical program. The following schedule pertains only to James.

MONDAY, WEDNESDAY, FRIDAY: WEIGHT TRAINING

- 3×12 parallel squats with 70 percent 1 RM (one-repetition maximum, or 70 percent of the maximum weight James is able to lift one time)
- 3×10 each leg split squats with 50 percent of body weight
- 4×8 inverted leg presses
- 4×8 push presses (front)
- 4×5 shrug pulls

TUESDAY: PLYOMETRICS

- 1×10 two-foot ankle hops
- 2×20 side-to-side ankle hops
- 2×20 hip-twist ankle hops
- 2×10 each leg split squat jump
- 1×6 standing jump-and-reaches

THURSDAY: PLYOMETRICS

- 1×10 two-foot ankle hops
- 2×20 side-to-side ankle hops
- 2×20 hip-twist ankle hops
- 2×10 rim jumps
- 2×20 single leg push-offs from a 12-inch box
- 2×20 alternating push-offs from a 12-inch box

WEEK 2

PREPARATION

Use resistance training to stress basic strength in the lower extremities.

PROGRESSION

Integrate higher levels of intensity into plyometric exercises to add complexity and intensity to resistance training.

PERFORMANCE

Remember that quality, not quantity, is the key in performing plyometric exercises.

WORKOUT SCHEDULE

MONDAY: PLYOMETRICS

- 3 × 10 front box jumps (18-inch box)
- 1 × 10 standing jump over barrier (36 inches)
- 3 × 3 double leg hops
- 2 × 10 rim jumps
- 3 × 10 two-foot ankle hops

TUESDAY: WEIGHT TRAINING

- 3 × 8 front squats
- 4 × 8 inverted leg presses
- 2 × 8 push presses (front)
- 2 × 8 high pulls

WEDNESDAY: WEIGHT TRAINING

- 5 × 5 back squats with 70 to 80 percent 1 RM

THURSDAY: PLYOMETRICS

- 3 × 10 side-to-side ankle hops
- 3 × 10 single leg push-offs
- 3 × 10 front box jumps (18-inch box)
- 3 × 10 rim jumps
- 1 × 5 standing triple jumps

FRIDAY: WEIGHT TRAINING

Repeat Tuesday's workout but replace the push presses with behind-the-neck push presses.

WEEK 3

PREPARATION

Emphasize heavy plyometric work. Use resistance training as a form of recovery.

PROGRESSION

Concentrate on building basic strength in those muscle groups associated with plyometric exercises for vertical jumping. Continue to build on both volume and intensity.

PERFORMANCE

Emphasize quality of effort by applying time and distance goals (for example, how quickly can the athlete accomplish 1×10 side-to-side box shuffles? How far can the athlete travel when performing standing triple jumps?).

WORKOUT SCHEDULE

MONDAY: PLYOMETRICS

- 3×10 depth jumps (from 18-inch box)
- 3×10 standing jumps over barrier (18 to 24 inches)
- 3×5 double leg hops
- 3×10 single leg hops with cone
- 3×10 side-to-side ankle hops

TUESDAY: WEIGHT TRAINING

- 3×8 front squats
- 4×8 inverted leg presses
- 3×8 behind-the-neck push presses
- 3×5 stiff knee cleans

WEDNESDAY: WEIGHT TRAINING

- 3×8 prone hamstring curls

  —Concentric: Raise weight with both legs.

  —Eccentric: Lower weight with one leg.
- 5×5 back squats with 85 to 90 percent 1 RM

THURSDAY: PLYOMETRICS

- 3×10 front box jumps (18-inch box)
- 1×3 standing triple jumps
- 3×10 lateral cone hops (12 to 18 inches)
- 3×10 alternating push-offs
- 3×10 rim jumps

FRIDAY: WEIGHT TRAINING

Repeat Tuesday's workout but substitute split squats for front squats.

WEEK 4

PREPARATION

Emphasize low-volume, high-intensity exercises. Neuromuscular preparation is directed toward maximal efforts with full recovery in both plyometrics and weight training.

PROGRESSION

The challenge is to work toward maximal efforts in plyometrics. Maximal vertical efforts with minimal ground contact time are a must.

PERFORMANCE

Resistance training as well as plyometrics should now be focused on power. The concept of maximal force applied rapidly is the key to developing vertical jump.

WORKOUT SCHEDULE

MONDAY: PLYOMETRICS

- 3×10 depth jumps (from 18-inch box)
- 3×10 standing jumps over barrier (18 to 24 inches)
- 3×10 single leg hops over cone
- 3×10 double leg hops

TUESDAY: WEIGHT TRAINING

- 5×3 quarter-squats
- 5×5 inverted leg presses
- 3×8 hamstring curls
- 5×3 front squats to push presses

WEDNESDAY: PLYOMETRICS

- 3×10 depth jumps to 24-inch or higher box
- 3×10 alternating push-offs
- 3×10 lateral jumps over cone (12 to 18 inches)
- 3×10 rim jumps

THURSDAY: WEIGHT TRAINING

Repeat Tuesday's workout but add 5×3 power cleans from the thigh hang position.

FRIDAY: RETEST

In our theoretical model of training the results of the retesting might look like this: To check for improvement, James is tested again on the tasks that he did at the beginning of the cycle. After implementing the four week training, James scores 22 inches for the standing jump-and-reach, 22.5 inches for the depth jump-and-reach, and 23 inches for the three-step jump-and-reach. As the training year continues, James should try to maintain his improved vertical jumping ability, and perhaps even increase it more. Future workouts will be designed according to his new goals.

LINEAR JUMP

The same five-step procedure for improving vertical jump applies to linear jumping.

STEP 1: CONSIDER THE ATHLETE

Connie is an 18-year-old college freshman with a mark of 36 feet in the triple jump. She has had high school experience as a triple and long jumper but has been average at best. She has no injuries or physical limitations.

STEP 2: ASSESS AND TEST THE ATHLETE

For improving linear jump, measure present ability with the following linear events:

1. *Standing triple jump for distance.* Connie stands on her preferred foot; then she hops, steps, and jumps into a pit. Measure the distance from the start of the jump to the landing.

2. *Five double leg hops for distance.* Taking off from and landing on both feet at the same time, Connie hops five times to see how much distance she can cover. Measure the distance from the start to the landing on the fifth hop.

3. *Flying 30 meters for time.* To measure the flying 30, the coach needs to mark off 100 meters on the track. The athlete gradually builds up speed over the first 60 meters. She is then timed between the 60 to 90 meter marks; this measures her absolute speed.

4. *One-repetition maximum parallel squat.* Connie determines the maximum amount of weight she can lift one time doing a squat in the same way that James did (p. 49).

5. *Five-repetition/five-second parallel squat at 60 percent body weight.* Again imitating the technique described for James, Connie attempts to perform five squats in five seconds.

Connie's test results will indicate her ability and readiness to undertake a high-intensity plyometric training program. Connie's scores on tests 4 and 5 show she meets the basic strength criteria. If she were deficient, it would be important to emphasize weight training for four to six weeks before undertaking intensive plyometric training.

Tests 1, 2, and 3 show Connie's present linear jumping ability and give data against which to measure her progress at the end of the program. Connie jumped 7 meters (23 feet) on the standing triple jump, covered 7.9 meters (26 feet) on the double leg hops, and had a flying 30 meters time of 3.4 seconds.

STEP 3: CONSIDER THE TIME FRAME OR CYCLE

Connie's program takes place over a four week period. The program has been condensed from a normal periodized training year to demonstrate the preparation, progression, and performance variables involved in program design.

STEP 4: SELECT THE TIME IN THE TRAINING YEAR

Normally a track athlete would begin training at the start of school in the fall. However, Connie will be involved in a crash course of training during the four weeks in February. She needs to prepare for the first outdoor meet that takes place at the beginning of March.

STEP 5: DESIGN THE PROGRAM

Plan each of the four weeks according to three variables:

1. Preparation
2. Progression
3. Performance

WEEK 1

PREPARATION

Use high-volume, low-intensity resistance training and low-intensity plyometrics to allow the body's soft tissues to accommodate to the stress of linear jumping and the impact of landing.

PROGRESSION

Emphasize variety in the type of plyometrics used, and review the skills of linear jumping.

PERFORMANCE

Concentrate on proper landing techniques and the use of the arms in performing low-intensity exercises. Make sure the concept of the amortization phase is understood.

WORKOUT SCHEDULE

MONDAY: WEIGHT TRAINING

- 3 × 12 parallel squats with 70 percent 1 RM
- 4 × 8 push presses (front)
- 3 × 8 lat pulls
- 3 × 10 each leg split squats with 50 percent body weight
- 3 × 8 hamstring curls
  —Concentric: Raise weight with both legs.
  —Eccentric: Lower weight with one leg.

TUESDAY: PLYOMETRICS

- 1 × 10 front cone hops (18 inches)
- 2 × 20 single leg push-offs (12-inch box)
- 2 × 20 alternating push-offs (12-inch box)
- 2 × 30-second segments of the 90-second box drill
- 2 × 10 front box jumps (12-inch box)
- 3 × 3 double leg hops

WEDNESDAY: WEIGHT TRAINING

- 3×12 front squats
- 4×6 inverted leg presses
- 3×10 incline bench presses
- 3×10 each leg split squats with 50 percent body weight
- 5×12 calf raises

THURSDAY: PLYOMETRICS

- 2×10 front cone hops (18 inches)
- 3×3 double leg hops
- 1×5 standing triple jumps
- 3×40 yards submaximal alternate bounding with double arm action

FRIDAY: WEIGHT TRAINING

Repeat Monday's workout but add three sets of 10 shrug pulls.

WEEK 2

PREPARATION

Weight training should emphasize work for hip adductors and abductors, as well as the hip flexors and hip extensors.

PROGRESSION

Many dynamic jumps should be done while moving across the ground.

PERFORMANCE

Linear jumping skill includes synchronizing arms with lower extremities to maximize efforts.

WORKOUT SCHEDULE

MONDAY: PLYOMETRICS AND WEIGHT TRAINING

- 3×10 front cone hops (18 inches)
- 3×5 double leg hops
- 1×5 standing triple jumps over barrier
- 3×40 yards alternate bounding with double arm action
- 3×8 split squats
- 3×8 lat pulls
- 3×8 hamstring curls
- 3×8 inverted leg presses
- 3×8 behind-the-neck presses

TUESDAY: REST

WEDNESDAY: WEIGHT TRAINING

- 3×8 lunges
- 3×8 high pulls
- 3×8 front shoulder raises with dumbbells
- 3×8 parallel squats with 80 to 85 percent 1 RM

THURSDAY: PLYOMETRICS

- 3×15 stadium hops
- 3×40 yards combination bounding with double arm action
- 5×5 barrier hops (hurdle hops)
- 3×5 double leg hops (for distance)

FRIDAY: WEIGHT TRAINING

- 3×8 lunges
- 4×6 lat pulls
- 5×5 inverted leg presses
- 4×4 high pulls
- 4×5 front push presses

WEEK 3

PREPARATION
Resistance training becomes more ballistic, with continued emphasis on performing lifts in positions similar to the joint angles reached in linear jumping.

PROGRESSION
Plyometric training becomes more complex yet is task-specific. Running speed is a consideration in this phase of training.

PERFORMANCE
Emphasis on plyometric training skills should be on distance, time, or both.

WORKOUT SCHEDULE

MONDAY: WEIGHT TRAINING

- 4×5 front squats to push presses
- 4×4 stiff knee cleans
- 5×3 inverted leg presses
- 4×10 split squat walk (exchange legs and move forward)
- 3×10 pulley weights hip flexion (to work on knee drive)

TUESDAY: PLYOMETRICS

- 3×20 stadium hops
- 5×3 double leg hops into 40-yard sprints
- 3×5 standing long jumps (for distance)
- 3×10 single leg hops
- 3×40 yards alternate bounding

WEDNESDAY: WEIGHT TRAINING

- 5×5 back squats with 90 percent 1 RM

THURSDAY: REST

FRIDAY: PLYOMETRICS AND WEIGHT TRAINING

- 5×6 multiple box-to-box squat jumps (18- to 24-inch boxes)
- 5×40 yards combination bounding
- 5×60 yards alternate bounding with double arm action
- 3×8 depth jumps to standing long jumps

Repeat Monday's weight-training workout.

WEEK 4

PREPARATION

Resistance training and plyometrics should now focus on power. Low volume and high intensity are the keys in both forms of training.

PROGRESSION

Single leg activities are of the highest intensity in plyometric training. Along with depth jumps, these become a vital part of development.

PERFORMANCE

Quality of effort will yield maximal distances in the shortest times during this cycle.

WORKOUT SCHEDULE

MONDAY: PLYOMETRICS AND WEIGHT TRAINING

- 5×20 stadium hops
- 5×5 barrier hops (hurdle hops)
- 3×50 yards combination bounding
- 3×40 yards single leg bounding
- 1×6 long jumps with a five-stride approach
- 5×3 parallel squats with 90 to 95 percent 1 RM
- 3×8 hamstring curls

- 5 × 3 inverted leg presses
- 3 × 8 overhead squats (snatch grip)

TUESDAY: REST

WEDNESDAY: WEIGHT TRAINING

- 5 × 3 power cleans from the thigh hang position

THURSDAY: PLYOMETRICS

- 1 × 10 depth jumps to standing triple jumps with slide-out landing
- 1 × 10 depth jumps to standing long jumps
- 5 × 40 yards alternate bounding with double arm action (timed with stopwatch)
- 5 × 30 yards combination bounding into sand pit

FRIDAY: RETEST

To check for improvement, Connie is tested again on the tasks that she did at the beginning of the program. After implementing this four week program, Connie scores 7.9 meters (26 feet) on the standing triple jump, covers 8.1 meters (30 feet) on the double leg bounds, and runs the flying 30 meters in 3.2 seconds. As the track season continues, Connie should try to continue to improve her linear jumping ability.

SAMPLE PROGRAM TO IMPROVE LATERAL MOVEMENT AND CHANGE OF DIRECTION

Once again let's apply the five-step procedure to develop a program for improving the lateral movement and change of direction abilities of an athlete.

THE TENNIS PLAYER

This program will allow Chris, at 13 years of age, the opportunity to develop movement and exercise skills that will help him accomplish greater strength gains once he has physically matured. Load or intensity of resistance is less of a priority at this stage of his athletic development. The emphasis is on developing core or trunk strength as well as lower and upper extremity strength. These need to be accomplished in order to improve his ability to move more quickly in a lateral direction on the tennis court. The plyometric drills are aimed at stressing those neuromuscular pathways that will also improve this skill.

STEP 1: CONSIDER THE ATHLETE

Chris is a 13-year-old tennis player with several years of playing at the Junior level, and has a sectional ranking in the top 10 players of his age. He has had little to no resistance training in his background. He has never been involved in a serious conditioning program prior to this.

STEP 2: ASSESS AND TEST THE ATHLETE

1. *Hexagon drill.* Standing in the center of the hexagon with his feet shoulder-width apart, Chris will begin jumping from the center across the front edge of the hexagon and continue around each side until he has made three round trips. He must return to the center after each jump to the outside and will be timed with a stopwatch from start to conclusion of the three cycles. Chris should be facing forward throughout the cycle of jumps.

2. *Twenty-yard sprint.* Chris will be timed in a 20-yard maximal sprint on a flat surface. This sprint can be conducted from a standing start position.

3. *T Test.* Using a T that is marked as 10 yards across the top with a 10-yard stem, Chris starts at the base of the stem and runs forward to the top of the T. He then shuffles to his left and touches a cone placed five yards away, shuffles to his right all the way across the top of the T (10 yards), then shuffles back to the middle. At this point Chris will backpedal back to the start. His total time is recorded.

4. *Medicine ball overhead throw.* Using a 4-kilogram (8.8 pound) medicine ball, Chris is allowed to take one step and use two hands to throw the ball from over his head as far as he can. The distance the ball travels from a start line to the point where the ball lands is measured and recorded.

The test results will once again dictate the type of program Chris is best suited for. This picture can be complicated by the fact that he is nearing puberty and has never strength trained before. Teaching the techniques of squatting, lunges, and other total body lifts will enhance the young athlete's abilities even though he is not lifting heavy weights. The load (amount of weight) lifted is not nearly as crucial in his development as is the need to learn skills of movement. Therefore, exercises should concentrate on submaximal plyometric drills that can be supplemented with strength exercises of high volume and low intensity (load).

Chris's results show that he records a score of 11.5 for the hexagon (60th percentile) and 3.2 seconds for the 20-yard sprint (70th percentile). On the T test, Chris had a score of 11.4 seconds, and he threw the medicine ball 16 feet.

These scores are typical of a ranked Junior tennis player this age. Because tennis is a sport so heavily weighted toward the skill of stroke production, athleticism is often overlooked, or secondary to the skills of the game itself. As with all sports, however, the rise of athletic ability of the participants is becoming obvious. Several articles have been published in tennis publications indicating that those individuals entering the professional ranks are becoming taller and heavier. This relates to the speed and force which can be applied during stroke patterns. Bigger and faster athletes are going to hit the ball harder, serve faster, and cover the court better.

The scores recorded indicate that Chris needs to improve in several areas of athletic ability. He needs to develop "start speed," lateral change of direction, and core strength as indicated by the short medicine ball throw distance.

STEP 3: CONSIDER THE TIME FRAME OR CYCLE

Chris is an example of a young athlete who is subject to the demands of a time-consuming practice and competition schedule. He really has no off-season. He doesn't participate in other sports and his school studies and tennis take up all of his available time. His slow time for tennis is in the fall between October and November.

STEP 4: SELECT THE TIME IN THE TRAINING YEAR

This program will be designed to fit into a six week period of time. It will consist of two weeks of a preparation period that will focus on improving core strength. The next two weeks will feature submaximal and low- to moderate-intensity plyometric exercises. Finally, the performance period should consist of two weeks of moderate- to high-intensity training, particularly for the lower extremities, that still take into consideration the age and abilities of this athlete.

STEP 5: DESIGN THE PROGRAM

Plan each of the six weeks according to three variables:

1. Preparation
2. Progression
3. Performance

WEEK 1

PREPARATION

Use medicine ball exercises to develop core and lower extremity strength. This time frame should call for high-volume, low-intensity resistance training. The most important criteria for this age is learning the skilled movements associated with resistance training. The age of this particular athlete will dictate the fact that the intensity of the resistance should be less of a priority.

PROGRESSION

Add exercises as tolerated, always aiming for a minimum of 10 to 15 repetitions per exercise. Resistance training for the young athlete should move from simple to more complex movements. The progression should also be from general to specific.

PERFORMANCE

Execution, execution, execution! The young athlete must be made aware of the proper positioning and movements of each exercise. Do not take anything for granted when working with this age athlete. Within the given attention span a lot can be accomplished to establish proper fundamentals of training.

WORKOUT SCHEDULE

Remember that with athletes this age attention span may become an issue. Try to keep the workouts crisp and moving right from one exercise to the next. Recovery is not as crucial in this type of athlete, especially when using lighter resistance aimed at developing a basic strength base.

MONDAY AND FRIDAY: RESISTANCE TRAINING EXERCISES

- 3×10 squats with 6- to 8-pound medicine ball (held on shoulders behind head)
- 2×10 split squats with 6- to 8-pound medicine ball (held on shoulders)
- 2×12 chest press with 10- to 12-pound dumbbells
- 2×12 pull-over with 10- to 12-pound medicine ball
- 2×12 seated rows (12 RM)

WEDNESDAY: PLYOMETRICS

Krumrie footwork pattern (p. 76)

- 1-2 for 5 seconds
- 1-6 for 5 seconds
- 1-2-5-1 for 10 seconds
- 9-8-5-9 for 10 seconds
- 1-5-7-5-1 for 15 seconds
- 9-5-3-5-9 for 15 seconds

Hexagon drill (3×3 circuits)

Two-foot ankle hop (4×10 yards)

Jump-to-box (12- to 18-inch box; 4×5)

WEEK 2

PREPARATION

Continue to emphasize basic strength and stability with the resistance training exercises.

PROGRESSION

Advance to more complex movements.

PERFORMANCE

Continue to emphasize proper alignment and relationships between each segment, trunk position, and tempo of exercise so that each is performed under control.

WORKOUT SCHEDULE

MONDAY AND FRIDAY: RESISTANCE TRAINING

Perform 3×10 repetitions for each of the previous exercises set up in a circuit pattern. Allow 30 to 45 seconds between each exercise for recovery.

WEDNESDAY: PLYOMETRICS

Krumrie footwork pattern

- 1-2 for 5 seconds
- 1-6 for 5 seconds

- 1-2-3-1 for 10 seconds
- 1-6-9-1 for 10 seconds
- 1-5-7-1 for 10 seconds
- 9-5-3-9 for 10 seconds
- 1-2-5-6-1 for 15 seconds
- 9-8-5-6-9 for 15 seconds

Two-foot ankle hop (5 × 10 yards)

Standing long jump (six reps)

Side-to-side box shuffle (3 × 30 seconds)

WEEKS 3-4

PREPARATION
Continue to build strength in such a way that the athlete learns to stabilize and control the body.

PROGRESSION
Introduce overhead lifting movements that force the athlete to control movements initiated with the legs and finished with the arms.

PERFORMANCE
Focus on initiation of a total body movement with the legs exerting force against the ground.

WORKOUT SCHEDULE

MONDAY AND FRIDAY: RESISTANCE TRAINING
- 3 × 10 push-ups (body weight)
- 3 × 10 front squats with 8- to 10-pound medicine ball
- 3 × 10 dumbbell presses with 8- to 10-pound dumbbells
- 2 × 12 lat pull-downs to the front (12 RM)
- 2 × 10 split squats (10 RM) each leg

CORE STRENGTH: MEDICINE BALL WORK (6- TO 8-POUND MEDICINE BALL)
- 2 × 10 trunk rotations (each direction)
- 2 × 15 pull-over passes
- 2 × 15 sit-up tosses
- 2 × 15 lateral tosses (each side)
- 3 × 10 overhead throws

WEDNESDAY: PLYOMETRICS
- 2 hexagon drills for time
- 3 × 20 seconds side-to-side ankle hops

- 3×20 seconds hip-twist ankle hops
- 1×5 standing long jumps
- 5×6 front cone hops (8- to 12-inch)
- 3×3 lateral cone hops (8- to 12-inch)

WEEKS 5-6

PREPARATION

Core or trunk strength should have a major emphasis at this point. Chris has been gaining in exercise skill and should now begin to experience actual physiological gain as well. One of the major demands of the sport of tennis is anaerobic endurance. The program should reflect this as a major goal.

PROGRESSION

Volume and frequency of exercise continues to rise in an effort to further develop strength as well as local muscular endurance.

PERFORMANCE

Exercises should move to become more specific to the sport so that the athlete can get maximum transfer from the weight room to the court. With the goal of improving lateral change of direction, the exercises should emphasize this area.

WORKOUT SCHEDULE

MONDAY AND FRIDAY: RESISTANCE TRAINING

- 3×10 push-ups (body weight) with three different hand positions (shoulder-width, wider, and narrower than shoulders)
- 2×12 lateral step-ups with 8- to 10-pound dumbbells
- 3×10 front squats to push presses with 10- to 12-pound medicine ball
- 1×10 lunges in four directions (front, 45-degree, side, and crossover)
- 3×10 dumbbell presses with 10 to 12 pounds

CORE STRENGTH: MEDICINE BALL WORK (6- TO 10-POUND MEDICINE BALL)

- 1×15 pull-over and touch toes
- 1×15 sit-ups
- 1×15 pull-over sit-ups
- 1×15 Russian twists
- 1×10 hip rolls
- 3×15 lateral tosses (each side)

WEDNESDAY: PLYOMETRICS

Perform a circuit of plyometric training using each of the exercises in weeks 3-4. Do five standing long jumps, then perform the hexagon, side-to-side ankle hops, hip twist, front cone hops, and lateral cone hops for 30 seconds each. Repeat this circuit three times, allowing 30 to 90 seconds rest between bouts.

COMPLEX TRAINING

You may have wondered by now whether weight training and plyometrics can ever be done in the same workout. Yes, they can—by athletes who are experienced in weight training and have also been through basic jump training. Early European writings labeled this combination complex training. Complex training occurs when you alternate weight training and plyometrics within the same workout session.

A recent study done by Lyttle, et al. (1996) at Southern Cross University in Lismore, Australia, has suggested that athletes who perform both heavy weightlifting and plyometric exercises "may enhance the use of elastic strain energy or facilitate the stretch reflex to a greater extent than does maximal power training." Maximal power training in this study consisted of doing jumps and bench press exercises on special machines designed to allow for maximal power development during these activities. Although this study did not look directly at combined or complex weight training and plyometric training, it did validate the use of combining these activities to achieve maximal results. No doubt more research in this area needs to be done; however, the theory tends to support the concept for performing exercises in this way.

One study conducted at the University of Utah by Adams et al. (1992), utilizing 48 male subjects, found that those who trained using a combination of squat exercises and plyometric exercises increased their vertical jump significantly (10.67 cm) over those who trained on squats (3.30 cm) and plyometrics (3.81 cm) alone, over a six week period. It was concluded that athletes who stand to benefit most from combined training programs are those competing in short-term power events. Among those included were track and field sprint, jump, and throw events; basketball; volleyball; alpine ski racing; and sprint events in cycling. It was also felt that when using a combined squat-plyometric program neuromuscular adaptations occur early in a training cycle (within the first four weeks) and therefore, one should be careful to avoid overtraining. This relates to the careful monitoring of the athlete's response to training intensity and sufficient recovery between workouts.

Combining strength movement exercises like squats with speed movements like the depth jump, double leg hop, or standing triple jump can be a very effective way to stimulate the neuromuscular system and provide variety for the athlete. The fact that there appears to be an arousal mechanism in the human body that is stimulated with maximal or near maximal lifting allows the athlete to take advantage of this situation when using plyometric exercises as well. There appears to be a short window of time when the body remains in the arousal or heightened state of excitement at the conclusion of a heavy set. By immediately adding a plyometric activity the athlete can take advantage of this physiological state and use it to perform better quality plyometric drills.

Combining the bench press with the power drop (a medicine ball exercise) is an example of upper extremity complex training. Other examples might include squats combined with hurdle hops. Lat pulls or pull-over lifts can be combined with variations of the overhead medicine ball throw. The use of the Romanian dead lift combined with overhead medicine ball throws from a glute-ham device are excellent combinations for developing low back and hip extensor strength.

In complex training, the volume of plyometric exercises should be reduced to a number that is easily workable between sets of the particular lift. For instance, an athlete might alternate sets of six half-squats with five standing triple jumps, then five double leg hops, then five depth jumps from an 18-inch box. This method of training can be used with any of the major weight lifts—squats, inverted leg presses, split squats, bench presses, power cleans, snatches, and push presses. As a rule of thumb, integrating two major lifts with plyometrics during a workout should yield maximum results. Trying to do any more than this usually requires too much time and brings the possibility of fatigue and overtraining.

Finally, remember that this form of training should always be preceded by a basic strength or hypertrophy phase of training. This type of training is an advanced form and works best and most effectively on the athletes who have a training base and history to fall back on. Execution of the lifts and the jump drills is extremely important and this is the wrong time to try to teach basic lifting techniques.

SUMMARY

1. There are four exercise variables to manipulate in accomplishing specific training goals:

- Intensity
- Volume
- Frequency
- Recovery

2. Plyometrics is a training method to be used with these other methods:

- Resistance training
- Anaerobic, sprint, and interval training
- Circuit training

3. A number of issues should be considered when developing a basic plyometric training program:

- The athlete's training level (determined through testing and assessment)
- The athlete's movement skills
- Time available
- The amount of plyometric activity to be included
- Training cycle length
- Safety

4. Vertical and linear jumping ability can be improved by carefully constructed, sport-specific plyometric training programs.

5. Complex training combines strength movement exercises and plyometric exercises to improve sport skills.

Rex Walters: NBA Basketball Player

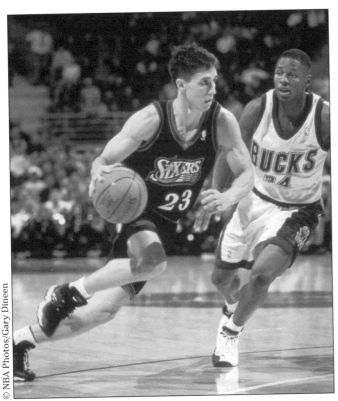

© NBA Photos/Gary Dineen

A point and shooting guard, Rex is a physically gifted athlete who used plyometric training to enhance his athletic talent. Able to jump to a 48-inch platform from a dead standing start on his initial evaluation, there was no doubt that he possessed a great deal of natural leaping ability. Plyometrics built upon his natural ability and helped him prepare for training camp. This is a crucial time for the professional athlete, since this is when he literally earns his job.

A typical plyometric workout for Rex Walters consisted of these exercises:

5 sets of 6 reps 42-inch hurdle hops (spaced approximately four feet apart)

6 sets of 3 reps 42-inch hurdle hops (spaced approximately 12 feet apart). This exercise requires the athlete to perform a standing long jump to an area just in front of the hurdle and then perform a vertical jump over the hurdle. Repeat for the entire number of hurdles.

4 sets of 10 reps depth jumps from a 42-inch box to a 42-inch box

Variations of the Frappier footwork patterns

5 sets of 1 rep standing triple jump

Keep in mind that this young man is a gifted, mature, and physically well-developed male athlete. He is a former All-American from the University of Kansas and has several years of experience in the NBA. He was able to tolerate this volume and high intensity largely because of his maturity and ability.

PLYOMETRIC EXERCISES

This chapter explains more than 90 different techniques that fall into the seven different plyometric exercise categories listed in chapter 2 (see page 14). For each exercise, you will be told what equipment you need, the starting position, and the action sequence required. The exercises within each category are arranged according to intensity level—from low to high.

The vision of what really constitutes a "plyometric" exercise has been bandied about for quite some time now. The term has been broadened to mean everything from 48-inch depth jumps to aerobic dance exercises performed on a "step." There have even been suggestions that plyometric exercises can be performed in a swimming pool. The East Europeans surely did not have this broad a scope in mind when the exercises were first developed. However, if one considers the parameters that go into describing a plyometric exercise, including the use of the "stretch" reflex and taking advantage of the elastic rebound tendency of muscle tissue, then the definition can be broadened to include many exercises that are plyometric in "nature." This definition allows for a broad range of activities to be included under the heading of "plyometrics." The purists of the conditioning world would have difficulty living with this definition but they would have a tough time arguing against it. Intensity of exercise is the key term. Plyometrics were meant to be maximal, all-out, quality efforts in each repetition of exercise. Anything less is not considered proper technique by those who would hold to an original concept of this type of training. The fact that differences in physical qualities of athletes can be affected by lower intensity training does not go unobserved. Young athletes who may not have the strength base or physical maturity to undergo the rigors of a maximal-effort training program can benefit by performing lower intensity drills designed to improve movement. The nature of these exercises can definitely qualify under the heading of "plyometric in nature."

One such program has been developed by the Acceleration Products company of Fargo, North Dakota. Largely the result of intensive study and meticulous planning by John Frappier, PhD, the program is growing in popularity throughout the United States with over 40 facilities up and operating at this time. Based on the use of "footwork" patterns and the "inverted funnel" principle, these drills have been carefully developed to fit with a high speed, intense interval training program on the "Super Treadmill." These drills begin with a fairly low level of intensity and increase in volume and intensity until they are finally used as part of a "complex" training scheme that allows the Acceleration Products group to claim decreases in 40-yard dash times and increases in vertical and standing long jumps of four inches and nine inches respectively after a six week training program.

THE INVERTED FUNNEL PRINCIPLE

This topic must first begin with a brief description of the body's center of gravity (C of G) and its relationship to stability and movement. The C of G represents a balance point, a location in the body about which all its particles are evenly distributed.

It is an abstract point that moves when the body segments are moved relative to one another. It is not even confined to the body. In the case of a "pike" position, it is possible for the C of G to actually be outside of the body. The C of G is most stable, or in balance, when the body is directly over the base of support, usually formed by the position of the feet relative to the ground surface. The wider the base, the lower the body's C of G in the standing position and the more stable is the individual. The standing C of G, in a practical sense, is somewhere in the vicinity of the belly button. The C of G will differ between individuals according to how their body mass is distributed. The individual with more mass or weight distributed through the legs will tend to have a lower center of gravity than those with thinner legs.

Having a high standing C of G is a distinct advantage to the high jumper. This is why you would want to recruit tall athletes to participate in this particular event. The higher the standing C of G, the less they have to work to get their bodies into the air and ultimately over a specific bar height. Shorter athletes must be very gifted in terms of muscle development and fiber types to have the explosive capability to reach elite level heights in the high jump. Regardless of the heights of the C of G, the athlete who can move quickly laterally and change directions easily is the one who has the skill to have the C of G move out away from the feet and then quickly recover. This moving of the C of G out from the feet results in a position of instability forcing the athlete to react quickly to recover their position or they will topple to the ground.

The concept of the inverted funnel is based on the fact that athletic movements require the individual to often move the feet out from under the body's center of gravity and then recover the position in a brief period of time so as to regain balance and stability. The essence of the Frappier footwork drills is that they teach the athlete to maintain the C of G in a relatively constant position while the feet rapidly work out from under it in all directions. The result is improved kinesthetic awareness, or that sense of where the body is in relation to the environment.

The purpose of this portion of the book is to present several different drills and to provide sample protocols. These protocols may be modified to suit the end user. The thoughts to keep in mind are that the metabolism of training for plyometrics in general is anaerobic. Therefore, these protocols are meant to be performed for brief time frames, and with a total volume of training in a range of 5-10 minutes of actual work with long recovery periods between bouts (five times the total work time).

ADMINISTERING THE FRAPPIER PLYOMETRIC FOOTWORK DRILLS

Frappier has set forth the following guidelines in carrying out this form of plyometric training. Due to the nature of the program, the Acceleration program sites as a group are collecting data on all of the athletes who go through the various levels of training. Therefore, they encourage "counting" each repetition performed during the course of any one exercise bout.

The general rule for all patterns is to count "one" each time the athlete returns to the starting point. For example, when executing a four square drill and going from box 1 to box 2, the scorer would count each time the athlete's foot or feet return to box 1. For the box 1-2-3 pattern, again, count "one" each time the athlete's foot or feet return to box 1.

When jumping foam barriers or boxes, the method of counting changes. Each individual contact with the ground or foot contact is counted. In the four square box 1-2 jumps with foam barrier, count "one" when the athlete contacts box 2 on the initial jump, count two when the athlete touches box 1 on the return trip, and continue in this manner for the remainder of the drill time. When using a box, count only the contacts with the floor or ground surface.

Another form of footwork drill in the Acceleration program is what is termed a "stride drill." These are drills featuring rapid exchanges of the feet in an alternating fashion on the top of a box. These repetitions are counted only when the support leg (defined as the leg which the athlete starts with on the top of the box) is pulled from the top of the box to touch the ground and then return to the top of the box. Thus, if the athlete begins with the left foot on the box, count one repetition each time the right foot touches the floor or ground surface.

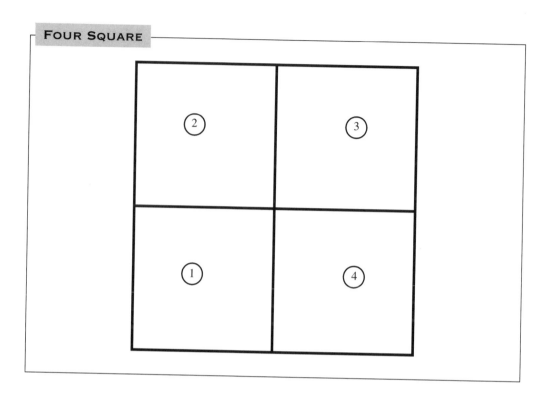

FOUR SQUARE

The four square plyometric pattern is made up of two lines 48 inches long crossing at right angles, forming squares 24 inches in each direction. Have the athlete start at square number 1 and jump in the order required.

When doing the program it is important that the athlete remain facing forward. The athlete should keep his/her center of gravity in the middle of the area that they are jumping in and only move their lower extremities from square to square as fast as possible. Each time the athlete returns to square 1 counts as one repetition. If an athlete's foot touches any part of the tape or they miss a square, the repetition does not count.

When called for, foam blocks 6 inches high and wide and 24 inches long are to be placed on the lines for the athlete to jump over. Center them on the lines separating each square in the direction that the athlete will be jumping.

When using three or more blocks together count the number of times the athlete touches the ground during the allotted time period. Each time the athlete knocks over the foam blocks, they must stop, reset the blocks, and start over.

SAMPLE PROGRAM

The following program is intended to be a representative sample of the jumps taken during a workout using the four square pattern.

Both Legs

    A. Box 1-2 Max. in 20 sec. _____

    B. Box 1-2-3 Max. in 20 sec. _____

    C. Box 1-3-2 Max. in 20 sec. _____

    D. Box 1-2-3-4 Max. in 20 sec. _____

Single Leg

  A. Box 1-2 Max. in 10 sec. R _____, L _____

  B. Box 1-4 Max. in 10 sec. R _____, L _____

  C. Box 1-3 Max. in 10 sec. R _____, L _____

  D. Box 4-2 Max. in 10 sec. R _____, L _____

Both Legs With One 6-Inch Foam Block

  A. Box 1-2 Max. in 10 sec. _____

  B. Box 1-4 Max. in 10 sec. _____

As with all of the footwork patterns presented, the above is just a sample program that can be reduced, expanded, or changed to fit the overall abilities and needs of the athlete. The user is only limited by his or her own imagination.

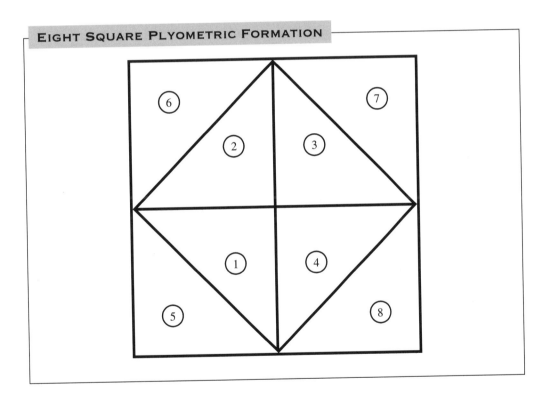

EIGHT SQUARE PLYOMETRIC FORMATION

The eight square plyometric pattern has the four squares from the first pattern plus another four lines added from each straight line at 45-degree angles. Each of these new lines is 24 inches in length. The numbering for the four new squares starts in the area of box number 1 with 5. Go up for number 6, across for number 7, and back down to number 8.

The rules that applied for the four square pattern also apply for the eight square pattern. Remember to have the athlete keep their body facing forward and to make sure that they do not touch any of the lines with their feet.

SAMPLE PROGRAM

Both Legs

A. Box 1-2 Max. in 10 sec. _____
B. Box 1-2-3 Max. in 10 sec. _____
C. Box 1-3-2 Max. in 10 sec. _____
D. Box 1-4-2 Max. in 10 sec. _____
E. Box 1-2-4 Max. in 10 sec. _____
F. Box 1-2-3-4 Max. in 10 sec. _____
G. Box 1-4-3-2 Max. in 10 sec. _____

Single Leg

A. Box 1-2 (2 sets) Max. in 5 sec. R _____, L _____ R _____, L _____
B. Box 1-4 (2 sets) Max. in 5 sec. R _____, L _____ R _____, L _____

Both Legs

A. Box 1-4-5-8 (2 sets) Max. in 10 sec. _____, _____
B. Box 5-8 (2 sets) Max. in 5 sec. _____, _____

Both Legs With Two 6-Inch Foam Blocks (place end to end along 1-4/2-3 lines)

A. Box 5-7 (2 sets) Max. in 5 sec. _____, _____
B. Box 1-7 (2 sets) Max. in 5 sec. _____, _____
C. Box 4-6 (2 sets) Max. in 5 sec. _____, _____
D. Box 8-6 (2 sets) Max. in 5 sec. _____, _____

Single Leg With No Foam Blocks

A. Box 1-2-3-4/1-4-3-2 (2 sets) Max. in 5 sec. R _____, _____ L _____, _____
B. Box 1-3 (2 sets) Max. in 5 sec. R _____, _____ L _____, _____
C. Box 4-2 (2 sets) Max. in 5 sec. R _____, _____ L _____, _____
D. Box 1-2-3-4-5-6-7-8 (2 sets) Max. in 10 sec. R _____, _____ L _____, _____

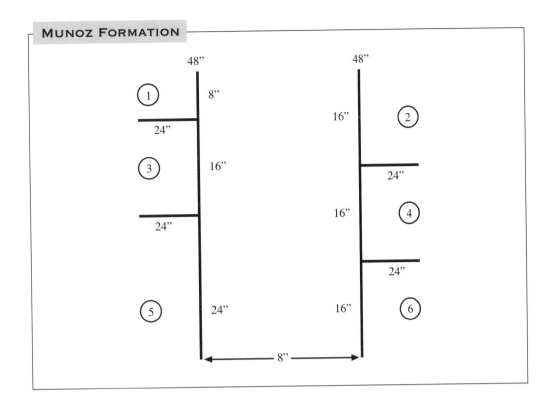

This pattern was designed for and named after Anthony Munoz, All-Pro offensive tackle of the Cincinnati Bengals. Again we use two strips 48 inches long laid on the floor 8 inches apart from inside edge to inside edge. The even numbered squares on the right hand side of the formation are 16 inches apart, separated by strips 24 inches long. On the left hand side, square number 1 is 8 inches, square number 3 is 16 inches, and square number 5 is 24 inches. On each of these squares the dividing line is also 24 inches long.

SAMPLE PROGRAM

Both Legs

   A. Box 1-2 (2 sets) Max. in 5 sec. _____, _____

   B. Box 1-4 (2 sets) Max. in 5 sec. _____, _____

   C. Box 2-5 (2 sets) Max. in 5 sec. _____, _____

   D. Box 2-3-4 (2 sets) Max. in 5 sec. _____, _____

   E. Box 1-2-3 (2 sets) Max. in 5 sec. _____, _____

   F. Box 1-2-3-4-5-6 Total Time _____, _____, _____, _____

KRUMRIE FORMATION

```
      3         4         9


      2         5         8


      1         6         7
```

This formation was designed and named after Tim Krumrie, All-Pro defensive tackle of the Cincinnati Bengals. This pattern resembles a tic-tac-toe board. Take four 48-inch long strips and lay out a pattern so that the inside measurement of each square is 16 inches along each side. Follow the pattern of numbering as in the other formations.

SAMPLE PROGRAM

A. Box 1-5-9 (2 sets) Max. in 5 sec. _____, _____

B. Box 7-5-3 (2 sets) Max. in 5 sec. _____, _____

C. Box 6-7-6-1 (2 sets) Max. in 5 sec. _____, _____

D. Box 6-1-6-7 (2 sets) Max. in 5 sec. _____, _____

E. Box 1-2-5-8-9-4 (2 Sets) Total Time _____, _____

Each of the above footwork patterns is designed to challenge the athlete's ability to move the feet away from the center of gravity of the body and become briefly unstable. Stability or balance is regained when the feet are once again under the body's center of gravity. This trains the athlete to move quickly and yet be aware of his position in space while performing the drills. This is known as kinesthetic awareness. These are challenging yet easily accomplished exercises that are designed to meet the criteria of utilizing the eccentric loading of the legs (stretch-shortening cycle) followed by concentric contractions so that they classify as plyometric exercises.

Lindsay Davenport: Women's Pro Tennis Player

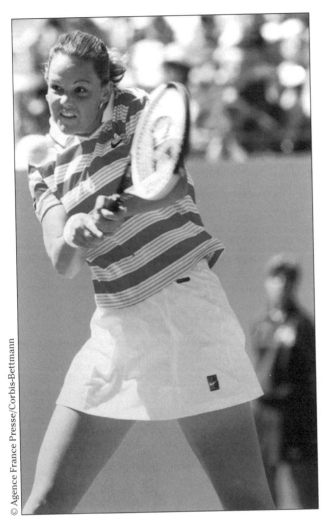

© Agence France Presse/Corbis-Bettmann

Lindsay, who has been ranked as high as second by the Women's Tennis Association, is a player whose prowess and powerful ground strokes are a foregone conclusion. However, her lateral movement and ability to develop speed within the first step have been subject to question. In the early days of her career this program helped her learn how to prepare to move quickly.

3 sets of 30 seconds single leg push-offs (12-inch box)

3 sets of 30 seconds alternating leg push-offs (12-inch box)

3 sets of 30 seconds side-to-side box hops (12-inch box)

4 sets of 5-5-5 squats with a 15-pound medicine ball

5 sets of 5 lateral cone hops (18-inch cones)

This program worked well for Lindsay as a female athlete whose physical maturity and leg strength were not quite fully developed. The goal was to improve response time to ground contact (quicker off the ground) and anaerobic endurance. This type of workout really helped to develop these two areas. Learning how to react quickly and maintain that performance for an extended period of time are essential ingredients for tennis conditioning.

Since turning pro in 1993, Lindsay has won many pro titles and was awarded a gold medal at the 1996 Olympics. At the 1997 U.S. Open, Lindsay teamed with Jana Novotna to win the women's doubles title.

KEY TO SYMBOLS

These drills are generally very safe and low in intensity so that they can be performed by athletes of all ages. However, as they progress in duration and difficulty they can be very demanding, even for the most elite athletes.

The symbols next to the exercise name show you what sports or activities can benefit most from that exercise and the exercise's intensity level. A key to symbols follows.

SPORTS OR ACTIVITIES

Baseball and Softball		Football	
Basketball		Gymnastics	
Bicycling		Ice Hockey	
Cricket		In-Line/Speed Skating	
Diving		Netball	
Downhill Skiing		Rowing	
Figure Skating		Rugby	

Soccer	Track and Field: Throwing Events
Squash/ Racquetball	Volleyball
Swimming	Warm-Up
Tennis	Weightlifting
Track and Field: Jumping Events	Wrestling
Track and Field: Sprints	

INTENSITY RATING

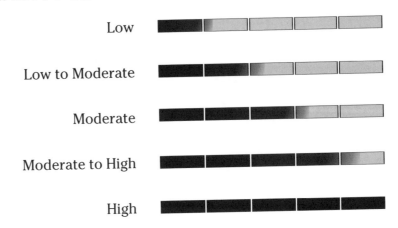

Low

Low to Moderate

Moderate

Moderate to High

High

Jumps-in-Place

Two-Foot Ankle Hop

Single Foot Side-to-Side Ankle Hop

Side-to-Side Ankle Hop

Hip-Twist Ankle Hop

Tuck Jump With Knees Up

Tuck Jump With Heel Kick

Split Squat Jump

5-5-5 Squat Jump

Split Squat With Cycle

Split Pike Jump

Straight Pike Jump

Two-Foot Ankle Hop

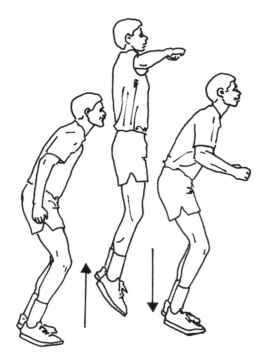

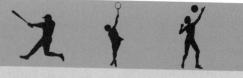

Equipment
None.

Start
Stand with feet shoulder-width apart and the body in a vertical position.

Action
Using only the ankles for momentum, hop continuously in one place. Extend the ankles to their maximum range on each vertical hop.

Single Foot Side-To-Side Ankle Hop

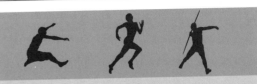

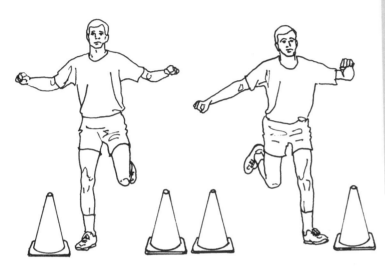

Equipment
Two cones placed three to four feet apart.

Start
Stand on one foot between the cones.

Action
Hopping from one foot to the other, land on the right foot next to the right cone, then the left foot next to the left cone. Continue hopping back and forth.

Side-to-Side Ankle Hop

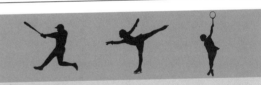

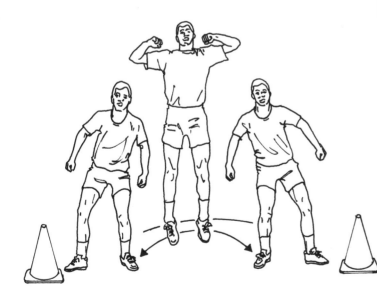

Equipment
No equipment is required, but cones may be used as borders.

Start
Stand with feet shoulder-width apart and the body in a vertical position.

Action
Using both feet jump side to side, covering a span of two to three feet; produce the motion from the ankles. Keep the feet shoulder-width apart and land on both feet at the same time.

Hip-Twist Ankle Hop

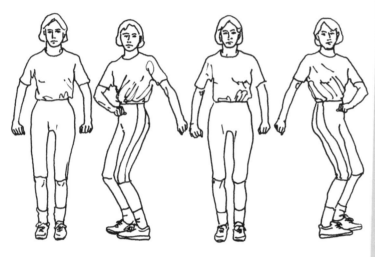

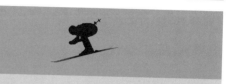

Equipment
None.

Start
Stand with feet shoulder-width apart and the upper body in a vertical position.

Action
Hop up and twist from the hips, turning the legs in a 180-degree arc. On the next hop, turn the legs to return to the starting position. Continue turning the legs from side to side on each hop. The upper body does not turn; the movement comes from the hips and legs.

Tuck Jump With Knees Up

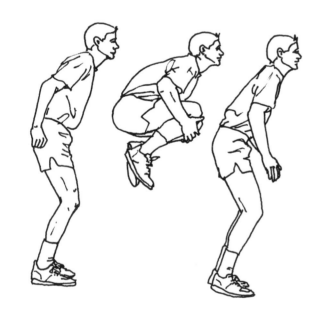

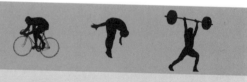

Equipment
None.

Start
Stand with feet shoulder-width apart and the body in a vertical position; do not bend at the waist.

Action
Jump up, bringing the knees up to the chest and grasping the knees with the hands before the feet return to the floor. Land in a standing vertical position. Repeat the jump immediately.

Tuck Jump With Heel Kick

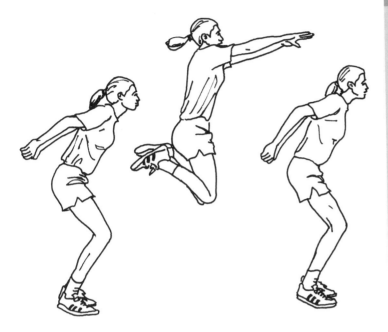

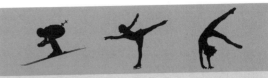

Equipment
None.

Start
Stand with feet shoulder-width apart and the body in a straight vertical position with arms by your sides.

Action
Keeping the knees pointed down (still in line with the body), jump and kick the buttocks with the heels. Repeat the jump immediately. This is a quick-stepping action from the knees and lower legs. Swing the arms up as you jump.

Split Squat Jump

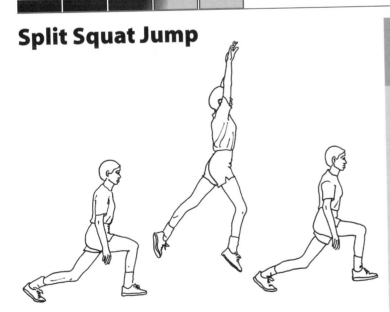

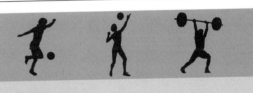

Equipment
None.

Start
Spread the feet far apart, front to back, and bend the front leg 90 degrees at the hip and 90 degrees at the knee.

Action
Jump up, using arms to help lift, and hold the split squat position. Land in the same position and immediately repeat the jump.

TIP Try for complete extension of the legs and hips when you jump. Remember that the ankle, knee, hip, and trunk all play a vital role in achieving maximal height while jumping and in speed when running fast.

5-5-5 Squat Jump

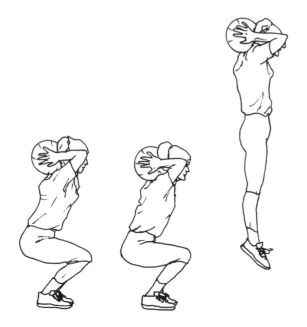

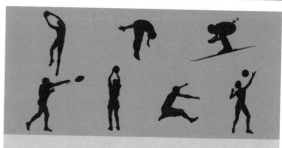

Equipment
Six-pound medicine ball or barbell with 60 percent of the athlete's body weight on it.

Start
Stand with feet shoulder-width apart and resistance on the shoulders.

Action
Perform five controlled squats to a thigh parallel position, then drop into the squat position quickly five times, then drop into the squat position and explode vertically five times. Maintain the weight in contact with shoulders throughout the jumps.

Split Squat With Cycle

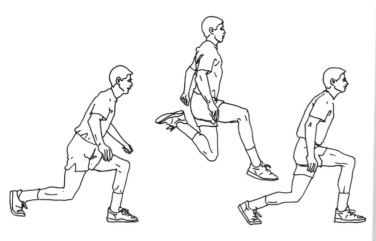

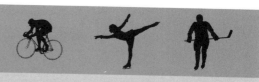

Equipment
None.

Start
Standing upright, spread the feet far apart, front to back, and bend the front leg 90 degrees at the hip and 90 degrees at the knee.

Action
Jumping up, switch leg positions—the front leg kicks to the back position and the back leg bends up and comes through to the front. While bringing the back leg through, try to flex the knee so that it comes close to the buttock. Land in the split squat position and jump again immediately.

Split Pike Jump

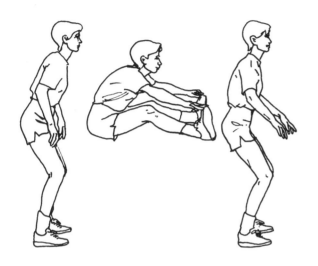

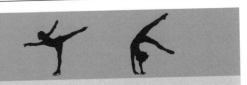

Equipment
None.

Start
Start with feet shoulder-width apart and the body straight.

Action
Jump up and lift the legs up and out to each side. Attempt to touch your toes at the height of the jump, then return to starting position. You should attempt to keep your legs straight. Try to keep jumps going in repeat fashion.

Straight Pike Jump

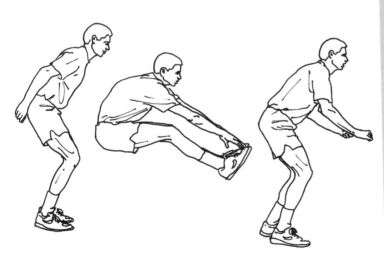

Equipment
None.

Start
Stand with the feet shoulder-width apart and the body straight.

Action
Jump up and bring the legs up together in front of the body; flexion should occur only at the hips. Attempt to touch your toes at the peak of the jump. Return to starting position and repeat.

Standing Jumps

Standing Long Jump

Standing Jump-and-Reach

Standing Jump Over Barrier

Lateral Jump With Two Feet

1-2-3 Drill

Straddle Jump to Camel Landing

Standing Long Jump With Lateral Sprint

Lateral Jump With Single Leg

Lateral Jump Over Barrier

Standing Long Jump With Sprint

Standing Triple Jump

Standing Triple Jump With Barrier Jump

Standing Long Jump

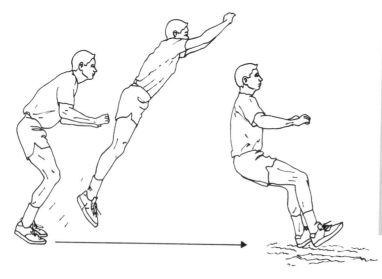

Equipment

A soft landing surface, such as a mat or sand pit.

Start

Stand in a semisquat with feet shoulder-width apart.

Action

Using a big arm swing and a counter-movement (flexing) of the legs, jump forward as far as possible.

Standing Jump-and-Reach

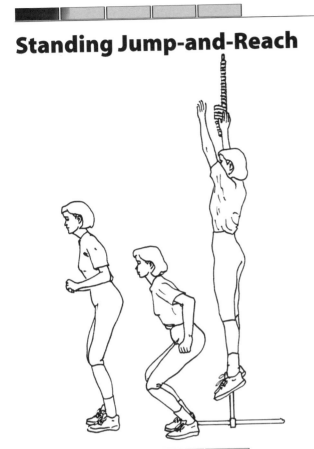

Equipment
An object suspended overhead, or a wall with a target marked.

Start
Stand with feet shoulder-width apart.

Action
Squat slightly and explode upward, reaching for a target or object. Do not step before jumping.

Standing Jump Over Barrier

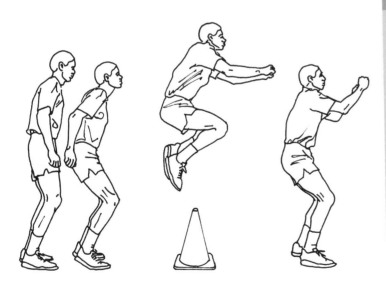

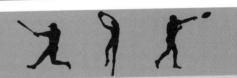

Equipment
One cone or hurdle.

Start
Stand with feet shoulder-width apart.

Action
Bending only at the hips, bring the knees up to jump over the barrier. Don't let the knees turn sideways or split apart to clear the object; the body should remain a straight line.

Lateral Jump With Two Feet

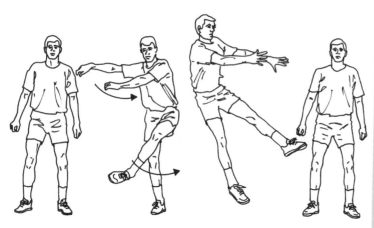

Equipment
None.

Start
Stand with feet shoulder-width apart.

Action
Swing the leg on the side to which you are going to jump across the stationary leg. Swing the same leg out to the other side and jump in that direction as far as possible, landing on both feet. Then jump back to the starting position by reversing the process.

1-2-3 Drill

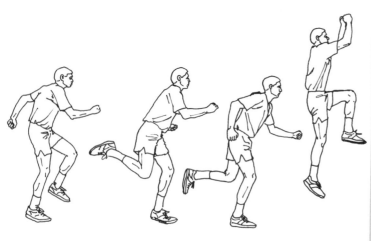

Equipment
A mark 40 meters from the start.

Start
Stand with one foot slightly in front of the other.

Action
Use three steps (left-right-left or right-left-right) in a continuous motion to simulate a takeoff. Complete the three steps with a quick-quicker-quickest rhythm, then explode vertically off the last one. Emphasize the action of takeoff and make the motion crisp. As soon as you land after the jump, step right into the next sequence of steps. Continue for 40 meters.

Straddle Jump to Camel Landing

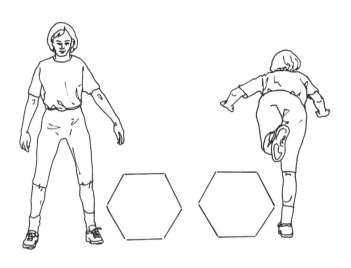

Equipment
A mat or flexible barrier.

Start
Stand with one foot in front of the other at an angle to the side of the mat or barrier.

Action
Using an action similar to a straddle high jump, plant the takeoff foot at an angle to the barrier and use a straight lead leg swing to lift the body over the mat. This turns the front of your body so it straddles the mat. Land on the foot that cleared the mat first, and let the trailing leg swing over and in a straight line behind you. Hold your arms out to the side for balance as if you were a figure skater on skates.

Standing Long Jump With Lateral Sprint

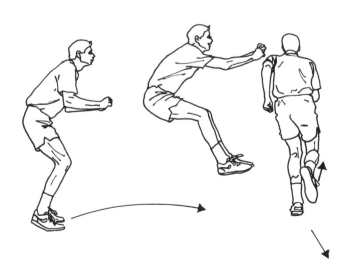

Equipment
Two marks, 10 meters to either side of a landing pit.

Start
Stand in a semisquat with feet shoulder-width apart.

Action
Using a big arm swing, do a standing long jump; land on both feet (try to stay up-right). Immediately sprint laterally (right or left) for three meters.

Lateral Jump With Single Leg

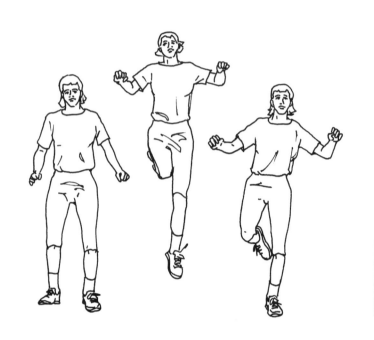

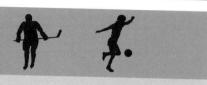

Equipment
None.

Start
Stand with feet shoulder-width apart.

Action
Jump up but push sideways to the left off the ground and land on your left foot. Immediately push off sideways to the right, landing on the left foot again. Continue pushing off from and landing on your left foot for the prescribed repetitions. Repeat this exercise using your other leg.

Lateral Jump Over Barrier

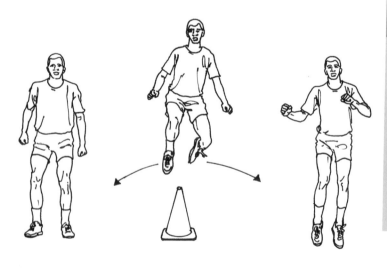

Equipment
One cone or hurdle.

Start
Stand alongside the object to be cleared.

Action
Jumping vertically but pushing sideways off the ground, bring the knees up to jump sideways over the barrier.

Standing Long Jump With Sprint

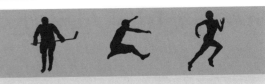

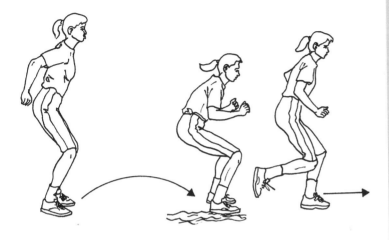

Equipment
A mark 10 meters from the end of jump and a mat, grass surface, or sand pit for landing.

Start
Stand in a semisquat with feet shoulder-width apart.

Action
Using a big arm swing, jump forward as far as possible. Upon landing sprint forward approximately 10 meters. Try to keep from collapsing on the landing; land fully on both feet, then explode into a sprint.

TIP Think "touch and go" when executing hops and jumps. You want to get off the landing surface as fast as possible.

Standing Triple Jump

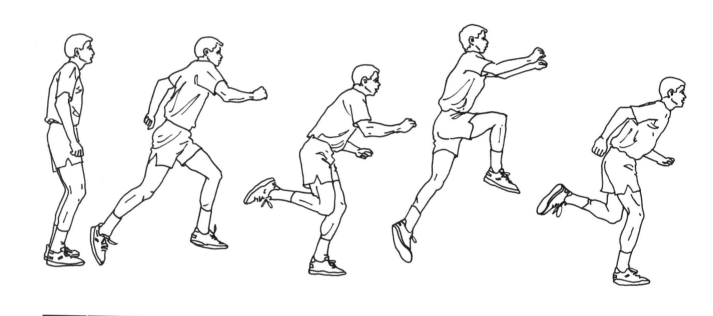

Standing Triple Jump With Barrier Jump

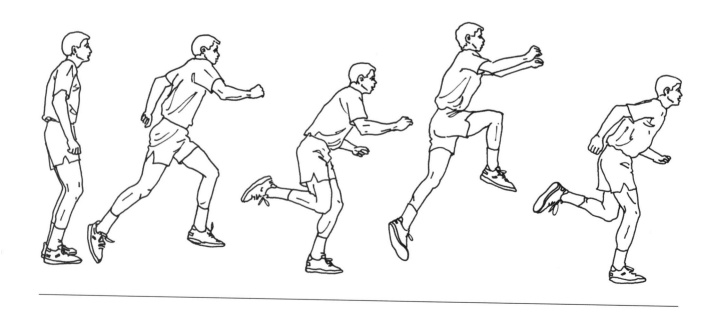

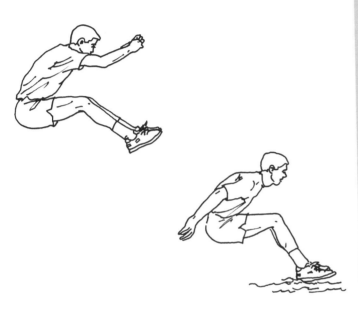

Equipment
A mat or sand pit.

Start
Stand with feet shoulder-width apart, three to six meters from a sand pit (distance depends on ability).

Action
Push off both feet simultaneously and extend through the hips to land on one foot (hop), then push from this foot forward to land on the other foot (step), then jump from that foot extending the feet forward as far as possible and landing with both feet in the pit or on a mat.

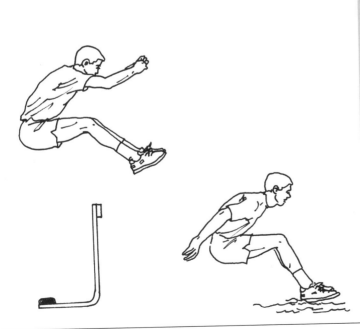

Equipment
A barrier (a line of cones or a mat) just in front of a sand pit.

Start
Stand with feet shoulder-width apart, three to six meters from a sand pit (distance depends on ability).

Action
Push off both feet simultaneously and extend through the hips to land on one foot (hop), then push from this foot forward to land on the other foot (step), then jump from that foot over the barrier, extending the feet forward as far as possible.

Multiple Jumps

Hexagon Drill

Front Cone Hops

Diagonal Cone Hops

Rim Jumps

Cone Hops With Change
of Direction Sprint

Cone Hops With 180-Degree
Turn

Double Leg Hops

Lateral Cone Hops

Barrier Hops (Hurdle Hops)

Standing Long Jump
With Hurdle Hop

Stadium Hops

Three-Point Stance With Single Leg
Hurdle Hop

Hexagon Drill With Barriers

Single Leg Hops

Wave Squat

Zigzag Drill

Hexagon Drill

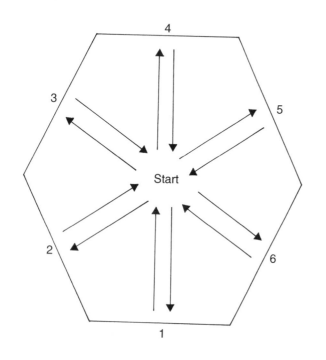

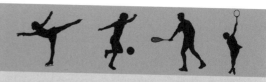

Equipment
A hexagon of tape on the floor, with sides about 24 inches long.

Start
Stand in the center of the hexagon with feet shoulder-width apart.

Action
Jump across one side of the hexagon and back to center, then proceed around each side of the hexagon. This may be done for a specific number of complete trips around the hexagon or for total time.

Front Cone Hops

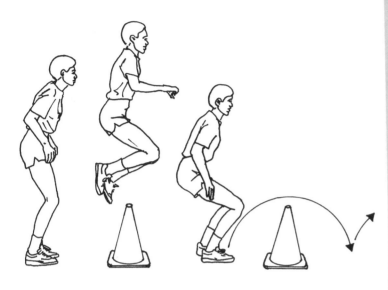

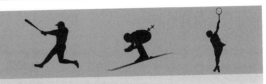

Equipment

A row of 6 to 10 cones or small barriers (8 to 12 inches tall) set up approximately three to six feet apart.

Start

Stand with feet shoulder-width apart at the end of the line of barriers (with their length spread out before you).

Action

Keeping feet shoulder-width apart, jump over each barrier, landing on both feet at the same time. Use a double arm swing and work to decrease the time spent on the ground between each barrier.

Diagonal Cone Hops

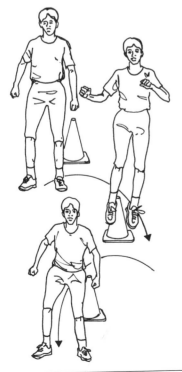

Equipment

A row of 6 to 10 cones or small barriers (8 to 12 inches tall) staggered approximately three to four feet apart.

Start

Stand with feet together at the end of the line of barriers.

Action

Keeping ankles together, jump in a zigzag fashion across the barriers, moving down the line. Land on the balls of the feet at the same time, and use a double arm swing to stabilize the body movement.

Rim Jumps

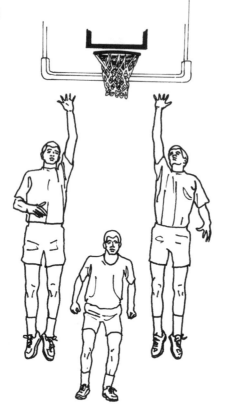

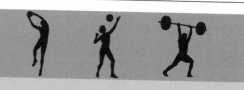

Equipment
A high object such as a basketball goal or crossbar on a football goalpost.

Start
Stand under the high object with feet shoulder-width apart.

Action
Jump continuously, reaching with alternating hands and trying to reach the object on every jump. Time on the ground should be minimal, with each jump being, at least as high as the one before.

Cone Hops
With Change of Direction Sprint

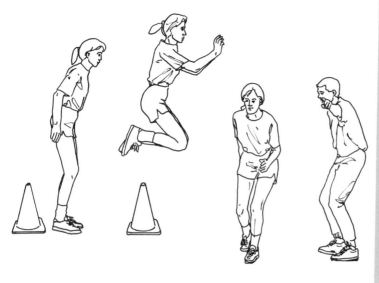

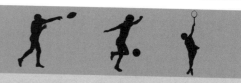

Equipment
A partner and a row of four to six cones placed three to four feet apart to form a Y.

Start
Stand with feet shoulder-width apart facing the first cone. Partner stands at the top of the Y, between the two spread cones.

Action
Do two-footed hops over the row of cones. As you clear the last cone, your partner points to one of the far cones. Sprint to that cone immediately upon landing from the last hop.

Cone Hops
With 180-Degree Turn

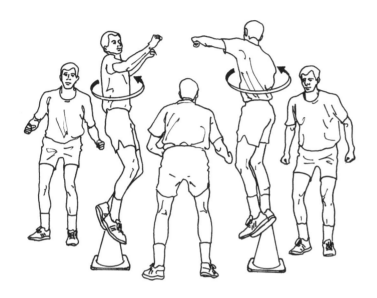

Equipment

A line of four to six cones spaced two to three feet apart.

Start

Stand facing forward, parallel to the line of cones, your feet even with the first.

Action

Jump. While in the air, turn 180 degrees, so that you land facing the opposite direction. Continue to jump and turn in the air down the entire line of cones.

Double Leg Hops

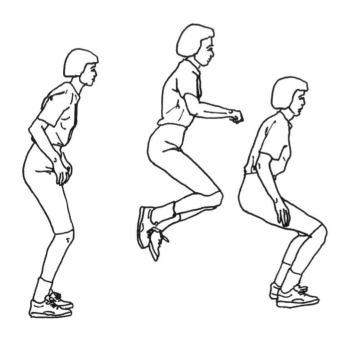

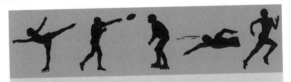

Equipment

None.

Start

Stand with feet shoulder-width apart.

Action

Squat down and jump as far forward as possible. Immediately upon touching down, jump forward again. Use quick double arm swings and keep landings short. Do in multiples of three to five jumps.

Lateral Cone Hops

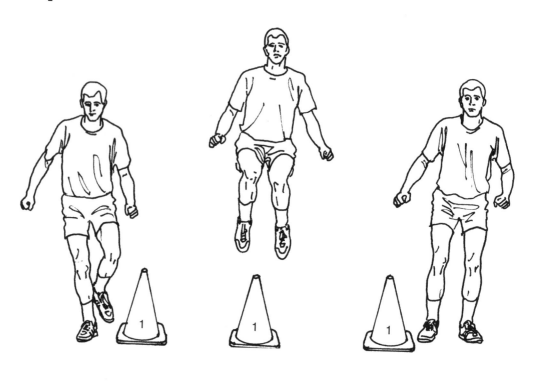

Barrier Hops (Hurdle Hops)

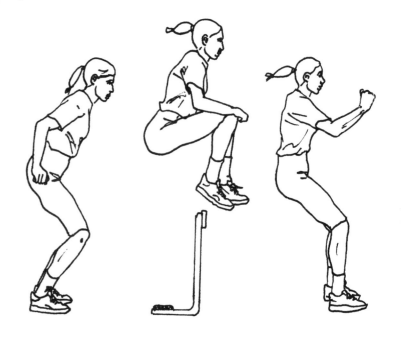

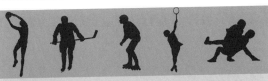

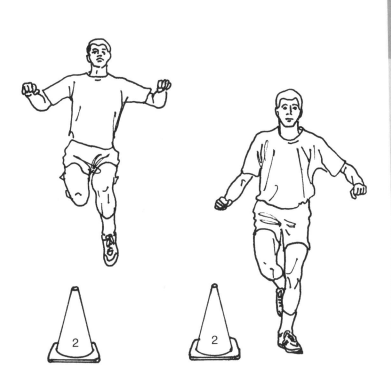

Equipment

Three to five cones lined up two to three feet apart. Distance depends on ability.

Start

Stand with feet shoulder-width apart at the end of the line of cones (with cones stretched out to one side).

Action

Jump sideways down the row of cones, landing on both feet. In clearing the last cone, land on the outside foot and push off to change direction, then jump two-footed back down the row of cones sideways. At the last cone, push off again on the outside foot and change directions. Keep movement smooth and even, trying not to pause when changing directions.

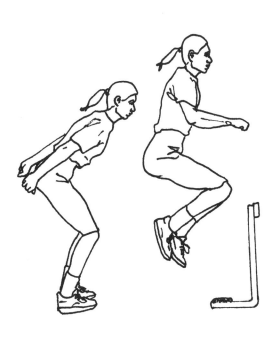

Equipment

Hurdles or barriers (12- to 36-inch) set up in a row, spaced according to ability. Barriers should be able to collapse if the athlete makes a mistake.

Start

Stand at the end of the line of barriers.

Action

Jump forward over the barriers with feet together. Movement comes from the hips and knees; keep the body vertical and straight, and do not let knees move apart or to either side. Use a double arm swing to maintain balance and to gain height.

Standing Long Jump With Hurdle Hop

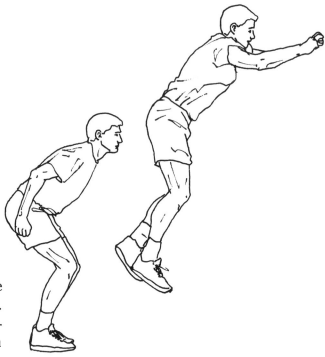

TIP Perform these exercises as if each jump is the highest and the best that you've ever done. Think of every effort as the "last" one. Maximal efforts in training make your efforts in competition look easy.

Stadium Hops

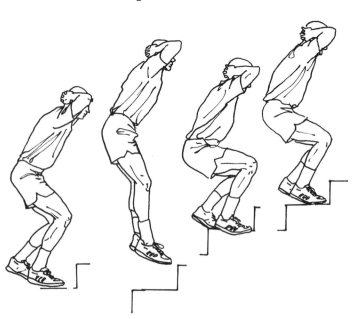

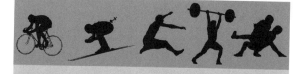

Equipment
Bleachers or stadium steps.

Start
Stand in a quarter-squat at the bottom of the stairs, with hands on hips or back of neck and feet shoulder-width apart.

Action
Jump to the first step and continue up for 10 or more jumps. Make landings light and quick; movements should be continuous up the stairs without pauses. Generally, the athlete should be able to take two steps at a time.

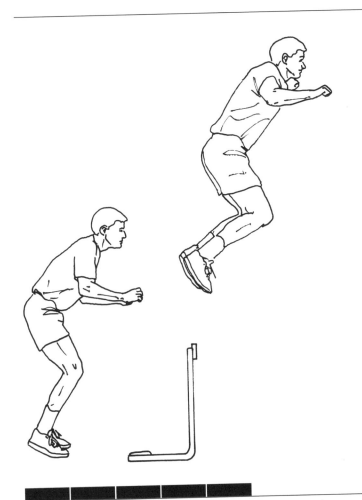

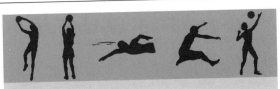

Equipment
Three to six hurdles 18 to 42 inches high placed 8 to 12 feet apart.

Start
Stand with feet shoulder-width apart in the ready position.

Action
Perform a standing long jump from a two-foot start. Upon landing approximately 18 inches in front of the hurdle, jump vertically over the hurdle. Continue moving forward over the remaining hurdles by repeating a standing long jump followed by a vertical jump over each hurdle. Use a double arm swing to maximize both the long and vertical (hurdle) jumps. Use hurdle heights that are challenging yet allow the athlete to perform the jumps by spending a minimal amount of time on the ground.

Three-Point Stance With Single Leg Hurdle Hop

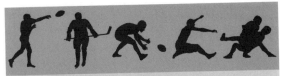

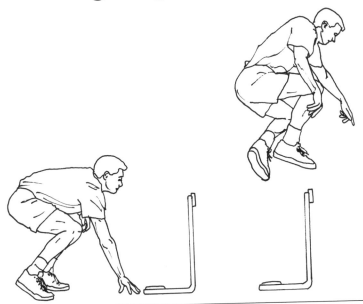

Equipment
A 12- to 18-inch hurdle.

Start
Assume a three-point stance position 24 to 30 inches in front of the hurdle.

Action
Drop quickly into a three-point or "down position" stance in front of the hurdle. Jump up and over the hurdle by pushing off of the "up" or "forward" foot. This requires the athlete to use a counter-movement of the front leg and develop drive power from it.

Hexagon Drill With Barriers

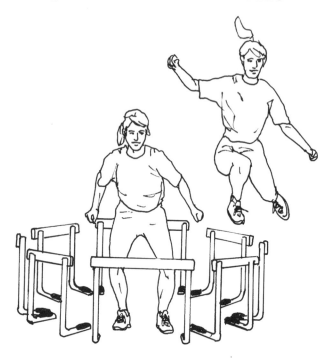

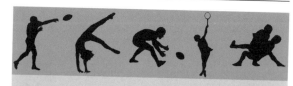

Equipment

Six barriers (6- to 18-inch hurdles) in a hexagon shape.

Start

Place barriers on the six sides of the hexagon. Stand in the center of the hexagon with feet shoulder-width apart.

Action

Jump across one side of the hexagon (over the barrier) and back to the center. Proceed around the hexagon, jumping the barrier on each side. This may be repeated for a specific number of cycles. Remain facing forward as you move around the hexagon.

Single Leg Hops

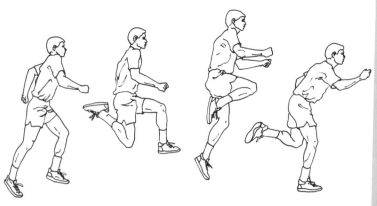

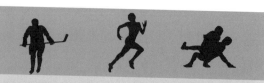

Equipment

None.

Start

Stand on one leg.

Action

Push off the standing leg and jump forward, landing on the same leg. Use a strong leg swing to increase jump length and strive for height. Immediately take off again and continue for 10 to 25 meters. Perform this drill with the other leg for symmetrical development. Beginning athletes will use a straighter jump leg; advanced athletes should try to pull the heel toward the buttocks during the jump.

Wave Squat

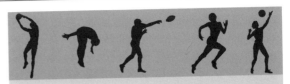

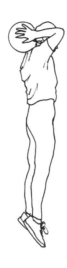

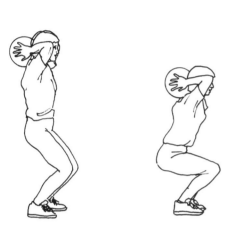

Equipment
External resistance ranging from 6-pound medicine ball to barbell with 60 percent of athlete's body weight.

Start
Start in a quarter-squat position with weight resting on the shoulders. Feet should be shoulder-width apart.

Action
Start moving forward by performing three double leg hops with the resistance on the shoulders, flexing the knees to approximately 130 degrees. On the fourth jump the athlete descends to a 90-degree position of knee flexion and performs a maximal vertical jump. Perform the sequence several times for maximal effort.

Zigzag Drill

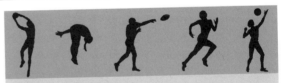

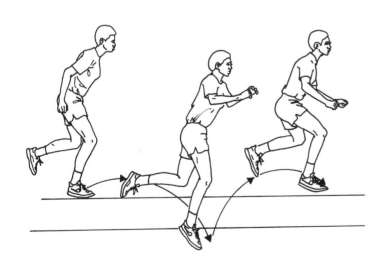

Equipment
Two parallel lines, 24 to 42 inches apart and 10 meters long.

Start
Stand balanced on one foot on a line.

Action
Jump from one line to the other in a continuous forward motion for 10 meters, always taking off and landing on the same foot. Do not "double hop" at the touchdown.

Box Drills

Alternating Push-Off

Single Leg Push-Off

Lateral Step-Up

Side-to-Side Box Shuffle

Front Box Jump

Lateral Box Jump

Multiple Box-to-Box Jumps

Pyramiding Box Hops

30-, 60-, or 90-Second Box Drill

Multiple Box-to-Box Squat Jumps

Multiple Box-to-Box Jumps
    With Single Leg Landing

Alternating Push-Off

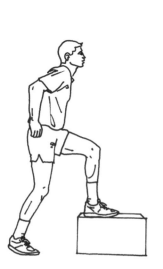

Equipment
A box 6 to 12 inches high.

Start
Stand on the ground and place one foot on the box, heel close to the closest edge.

Action
Push off of the foot on the box to gain as much height as possible by extending through the entire leg and foot; land with feet reversed (the box foot lands a split second before the ground foot). Use a double arm swing for height and balance.

Single Leg Push-Off

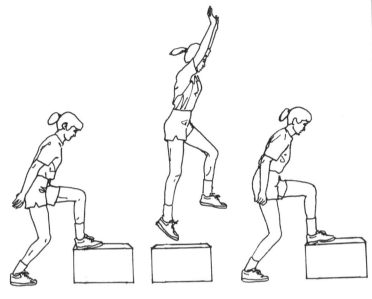

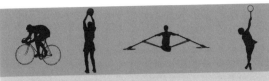

Equipment
A box 6 to 12 inches high.

Start
Stand on the ground and place one foot on the box, heel close to the closest edge.

Action
Push off of the foot on top of the box to gain as much height as possible by extending through the entire leg and foot. Land with the same foot on top of the box and push off again. Use a double arm swing for height and balance.

Lateral Step-Up

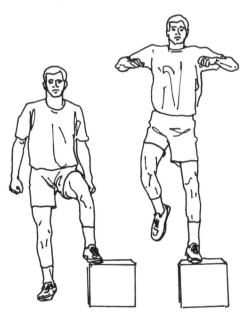

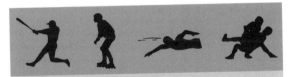

Equipment
A box 6 to 12 inches high.

Start
Standing to the side of the box, place the foot closest to the box on top.

Action
Use the leg on the box to raise the body until the leg is extended, then lower to starting position. Don't push off the foot on the ground; use the bent leg to do all the work. Perform exercise using both legs.

Side-to-Side Box Shuffle

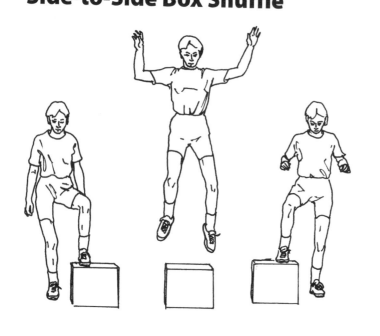

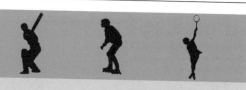

Equipment
A box 12 to 24 inches high.

Start
Stand to one side of the box with the left foot raised onto the middle of the box.

Action
Using a double arm swing, jump up and over to the other side of the box, landing with the right foot on top of the box and the left foot on the floor. This drill should be done in a continuous motion, shuffling back and forth across the top of the box.

Front Box Jump

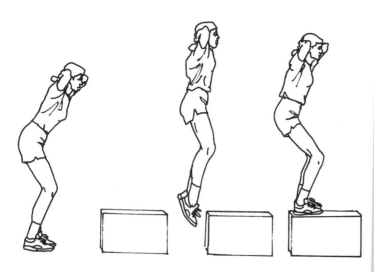

Equipment
A box (height 12 to 42 inches depending on ability).

Start
Stand facing the box with feet shoulder-width apart and hands behind the head.

Action
Jump up and land softly with both feet on the box. Step back down and repeat. For a more advanced exercise, hop down from the box and immediately jump back onto it. Use a variety of box heights, starting with 12-inch boxes and building up to 42 inches with time.

Lateral Box Jump

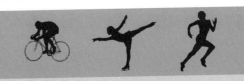

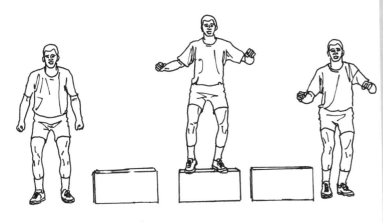

Equipment
A single box (or a row of three to five boxes) 12 to 42 inches high.

Start
Stand at the side of the box with feet shoulder-width apart.

Action
Jump onto the box and back to the ground on the other side. The exercise can be done as a single or as continuous movement across a line of three to five boxes of the same height (jumping to the ground between boxes).

Multiple Box-to-Box Jumps

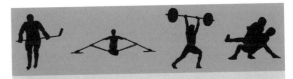

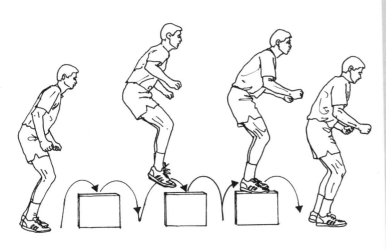

Equipment
Three to five boxes of the same height placed in a row (box height according to ability).

Start
Stand with feet shoulder-width apart at the end of the row of boxes (with their length spread out before you).

Action
Jump onto the first box, then off on the other side, onto the second box, then off, and so on down the row. After jumping off the last box, walk back to the start for recovery.

Pyramiding Box Hops

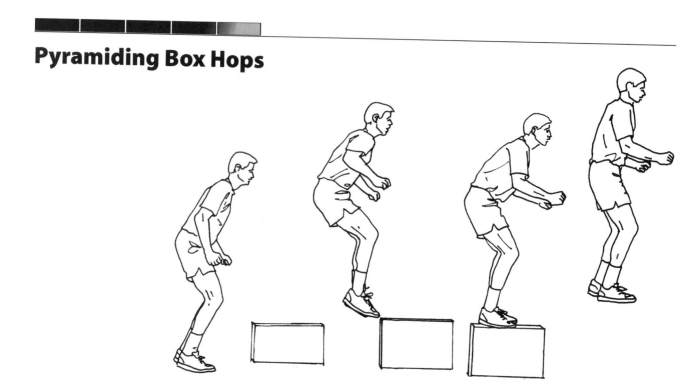

| 30 s | 60 s | 90 s |

30-, 60-, or 90-Second Box Drill

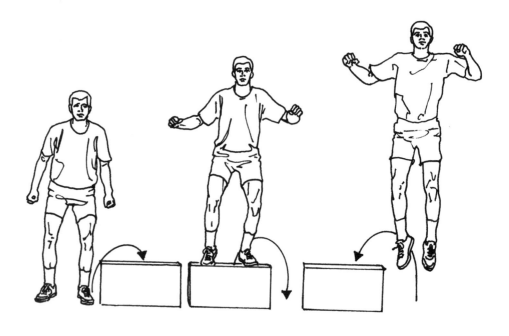

TIP In order to learn to react faster to ground contact, visualize the ground being "hot." You want to spend as little time as you can on the hot surface.

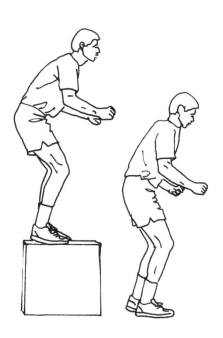

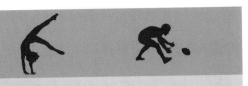

Equipment

Three to five boxes of increasing height, evenly spaced two to three feet apart.

Start

Stand with feet shoulder-width apart looking down the row of boxes.

Action

Jump onto the first box, then off on the other side, onto the second box, then off, and so on down the row. Walk back to the start after finishing the sequence for recovery, or immediately hop back down the row of boxes.

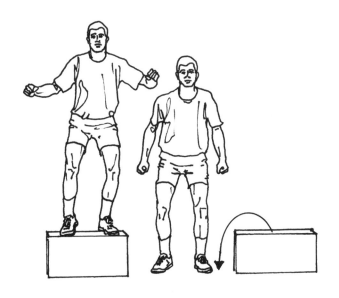

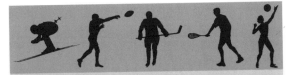

Equipment

A box 12 inches high, 20 inches wide, and 30 inches deep.

Start

Stand at the side of the box with feet shoulder-width apart.

Action

Jump onto the box, back to the ground on the other side, then back onto the box. Continue to jump across the top of the box for an allotted time, with each touch on top of the box counting as one. Use the following guidelines:

- 30 touches in 30 seconds—Start of training (low intensity)
- 60 touches in 60 seconds—Start of season (moderate intensity)
- 90 touches in 90 seconds—Championship season (high intensity)

Multiple Box-to-Box Squat Jumps

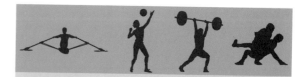

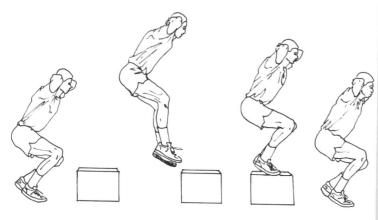

Equipment

A row of boxes of the same height (box height according to ability).

Start

Stand in a deep-squat position with feet shoulder-width apart looking down the row of boxes, hands clasped behind the head.

Action

Jump to the first box, landing softly in a squat position. Maintaining the squat position, jump off the box on the other side and immediately onto and off of the following boxes. Keep hands on the hips or behind the head.

Multiple Box-to-Box Jumps With Single Leg Landing

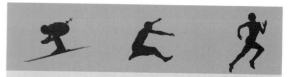

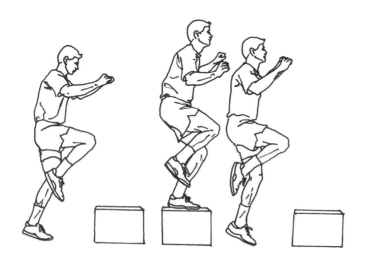

Equipment

A row of boxes 6 to 12 inches high. Increase height to 18 to 24 inches after a period of time.

Start

Stand on one foot looking down the row of boxes.

Action

Jump onto the first box, landing on the takeoff foot, then jump to the floor, landing on the same foot. Continue in this fashion down the row of boxes. Repeat the exercise using the other leg. This is a strenuous exercise; the athlete must be in top form, and strict concentration is needed to prevent injury.

Depth Jumps

Jump From Box

Jump to Box

Step-Close Jump-and-Reach

Depth Jump

Depth Jump to Prescribed Height

Incline Push-Up Depth Jump

Squat Depth Jump

Depth Jump With 180-Degree Turn

Depth Jump With 360-Degree Turn

Depth Jump to Rim Jump

Single Leg Depth Jump

Depth Jump With Lateral Movement

Depth Jump With Stuff

Depth Jump With Blocking Bag

Depth Jump With Pass Catching

Depth Jump With Backward Glide

Handstand Depth Jump

Depth Jump Over Barrier

Depth Jump to Standing Long Jump

Jump From Box

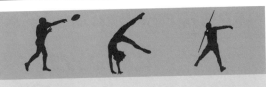

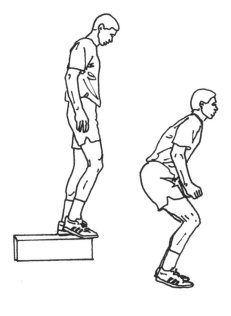

Equipment
A box 6 to 18 inches high.

Start
Stand on the box with feet shoulder-width apart.

Action
Squat slightly and step from the box and drop to the floor. Attempt to quickly absorb the landing and "freeze" as soon as contact is made with the ground.

Jump to Box

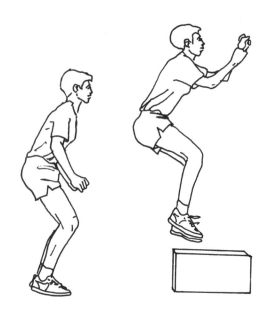

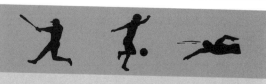

Equipment

A box 6 to 12 inches high with a top surface no smaller than 24 inches square.

Start

Stand on the ground with feet shoulder-width apart, facing a box.

Action

Squat slightly and, using the double arm swing, jump from the ground onto the box.

Step-Close Jump-and-Reach

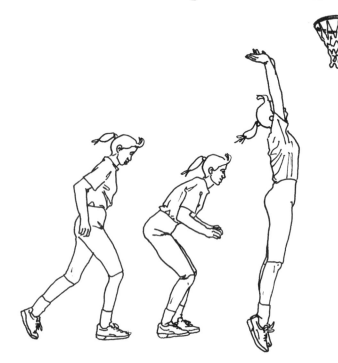

Equipment

An object suspended at the peak of the athlete's jump.

Start

Stand in a staggered stance front to back.

Action

Take a short step forward with the preferred foot and quickly bring the back foot together with the front foot (a step-close technique). Then jump vertically, reaching for the suspended object.

Depth Jump

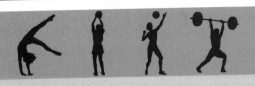

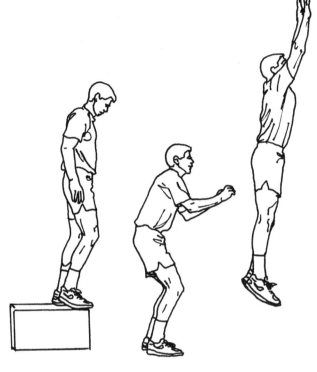

Equipment
A box 12 inches high.

Start
Stand on the box, toes close to the front edge.

Action
Step from the box and drop to land on both feet. Try to anticipate the landing and spring up as quickly as you can. Keep the body from "settling" on the landing, and make the ground contact as short as possible.

Depth Jump to Prescribed Height

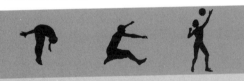

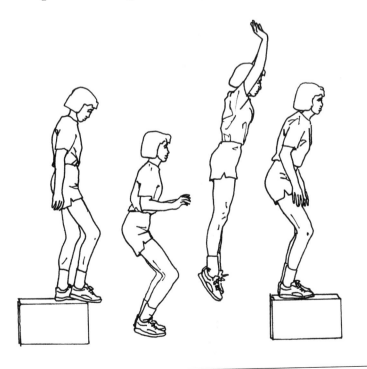

Equipment
Two boxes of equal height placed two to four feet apart. Height and distance depend on ability.

Start
Stand on one box, toes close to the front edge and feet shoulder-width apart, facing the second box.

Action
Step off the box, landing on both feet, and jump onto the second box, landing lightly. The jump from the ground should be as quick as possible.

Incline Push-Up Depth Jump

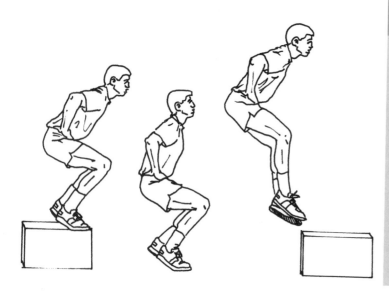

> **TIP** The body has a way of setting itself for action, so mentally prepare yourself for "contact." By thinking about what is going to happen when you contact the ground, you are mentally readying yourself for action. This "presets" or "biases" the muscle for action.

Squat Depth Jump

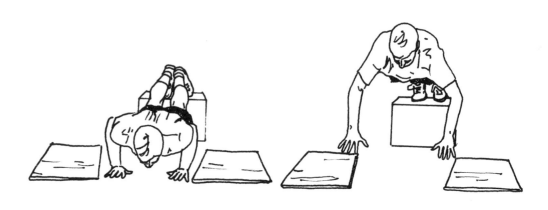

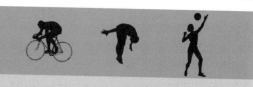

Equipment
One or two boxes 12 to 42 inches high.

Start
Stand on a box in a quarter- to half-squat, toes close to the edge.

Action
Step off the box and land in a 90-degree squat position. Explode up out of the squat and land solidly in a squat. For added difficulty, land on a second box of equal height after doing the jump.

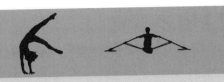

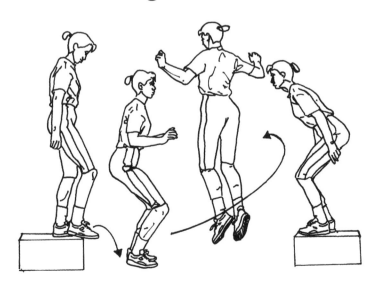

Equipment

Two mats, three to four inches high, placed shoulder-width apart, and a box high enough to elevate the athlete's feet above the shoulders when the athlete is in a push-up position.

Start

Face the floor as if you were going to do a push-up, with your feet on the box and your hands between the mats.

Action

Push off the ground with your hands and land with one hand on each mat. Either remove one hand at a time from the mats and place them in the starting position or, for added difficulty, push off the mats with both hands and catch yourself in the starting position.

Depth Jump
With 180-Degree Turn

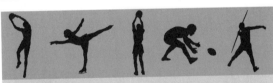

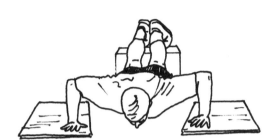

Equipment

One or two boxes 12 to 42 inches high.

Start

Stand on a box, toes close to the edge.

Action

Step off the box and land on both feet. Immediately jump up and do a 180-degree turn in the air, landing again on both feet. For added difficulty, land on a second box after doing the turn.

Depth Jump
With 360-Degree Turn

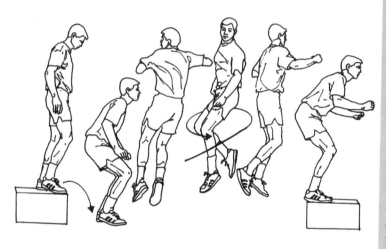

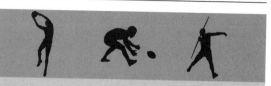

Equipment
One or two boxes 12 to 42 inches high.

Start
Stand on a box, toes close to the edge.

Action
Step off the box and land on both feet. Immediately jump up and do a 360-degree turn in the air, landing again on both feet. For added difficulty, land on a second box after doing the turn. This is an advanced drill—it should not be performed by beginners.

Depth Jump to Rim Jump

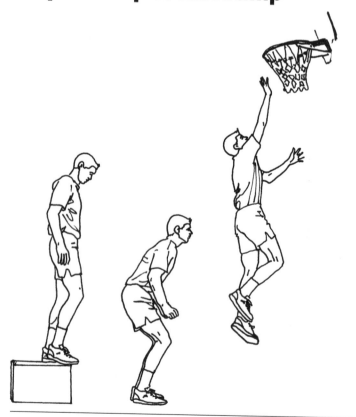

Equipment
A box 12 to 42 inches high placed in front of an elevated marker (such as a basketball hoop).

Start
Stand on the box, toes close to the edge and facing the high object.

Action
Step off the box and land on both feet. Immediately jump up, reaching with one hand toward the marker, and then do repeated jumps, alternating hands and trying to reach the object each time. Time on the ground should be very short, with each jump being as high as the one before. Perform three to five rim jumps after each depth jump.

Single Leg Depth Jump

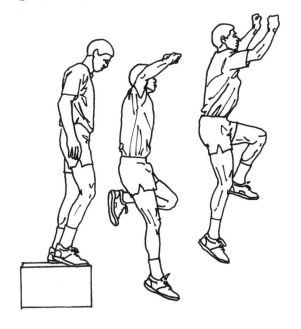

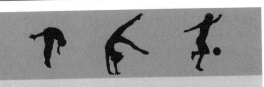

Equipment
A box 12 to 18 inches high.

Start
Stand on the box, toes close to the edge.

Action
Step off the box and land on one foot. Then jump as high as possible, landing on the same foot. Keep the ground contact as short as possible. For added difficulty, jump to a second box after the jump. This is an advanced drill; it should not be performed by beginners.

Depth Jump With Lateral Movement

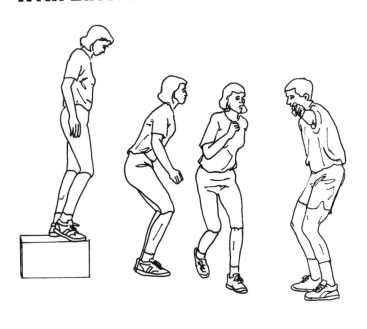

Equipment
A partner and a box 12 to 42 inches high.

Start
Stand on the box, toes close to the edge, facing your partner.

Action
Step off the box and land on both feet. As you land, your partner points to the right or left; sprint in that direction for 10 to 12 meters.

Depth Jump With Stuff

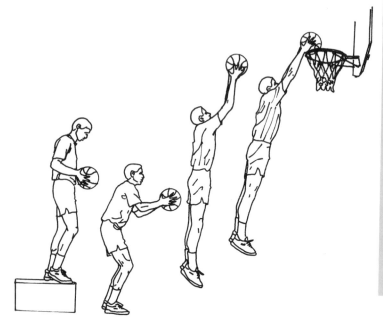

Equipment
A box 12 to 42 inches high, a basketball, and a basketball goal.

Start
Stand on the box, toes close to the edge, holding a ball in front of you.

Action
Step off the box and land on both feet. Explode up and forward while extending your arms and the ball up. Try to stuff the ball in the basket, or at least to touch the rim.

Depth Jump With Blocking Bag

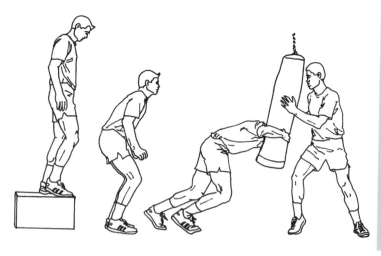

Equipment
A box 12 to 42 inches high and a partner with a blocking bag.

Start
Stand on the box, toes close to the edge. The partner stands facing the box, about four feet away.

Action
Step off the box and land on both feet. Upon landing, explode into the blocking bag shoulder first.

Depth Jump With Pass Catching

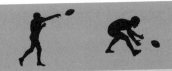

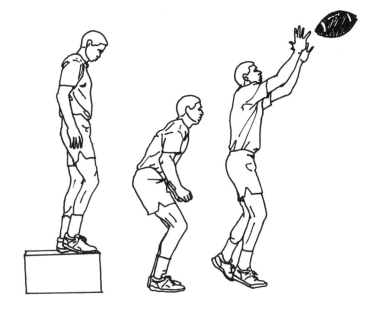

Equipment

A box 12 to 42 inches high and a partner with a football.

Start

Stand on the box, toes close to the edge, facing your partner.

Action

Step off the box and land on both feet. Explode up and forward, extending your arms to catch a pass from your partner at the peak of your jump.

Depth Jump
With Backward Glide

Equipment

A box 12 to 42 inches high.

Start

Stand with heels close to the back of the box and with feet shoulder-width apart.

Action

Step backward off the box and land on both feet. Immediately upon landing, thrust one leg back and perform a glide pattern step as if shot putting.

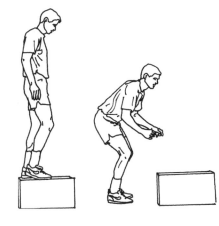

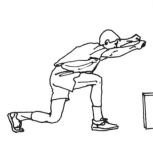

Handstand Depth Jump

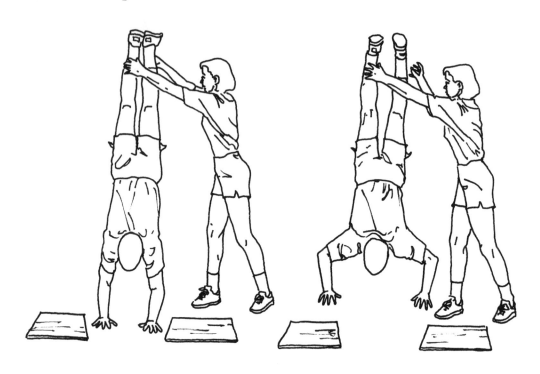

Depth Jump Over Barrier

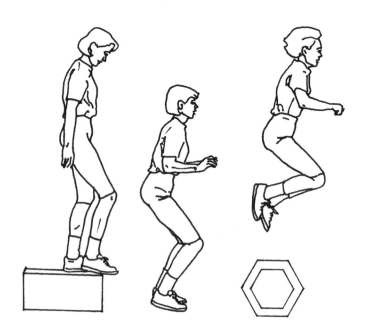

Equipment
A 12- to 42-inch box and a barrier 28 to 36 inches high, placed about three feet from the box.

Start
Stand on the box with feet shoulder-width apart.

Action
Step off the box and, upon landing, jump over the barrier.

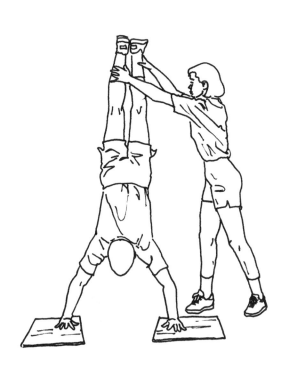

Equipment
A partner and two mats or padded boxes, three to four inches high, placed shoulder-width apart.

Start
Stand between the mats or padded boxes, with a partner standing behind, and do a handstand on the floor.

Action
Push off the floor with the hands, landing with one hand on each mat. Then push up off the mats and land with your hands in their starting positions. The partner spots for the athlete, ensuring that the body stays vertical.

Depth Jump to Standing Long Jump

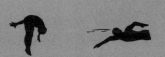

Equipment
A box 12 to 42 inches high.

Start
Stand on the box, feet shoulder-width apart and toes close to the edge.

Action
Step off the box and land on both feet. Immediately upon landing, jump as far forward as possible, again landing on both feet.

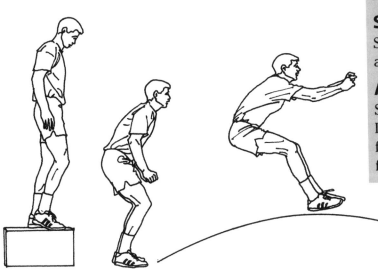

Bounding

Skipping

Power Skipping

Backward Skipping

Side Skipping With Big Arm Swing

Moving Split Squat With Cycle

Alternate Bounding
With Single Arm Action

Alternate Bounding
With Double Arm Action

Combination Bounding
With Single Arm Action

Combination Bounding
With Double Arm Action

Combination Bounding
With Vertical Jump

Single Leg Bounding

TIP Remember that with an arm swing, long (straight) arms generate force, short (bent) arms generate speed. Examine your sport or event and see which one is most beneficial for you to use.

Skipping

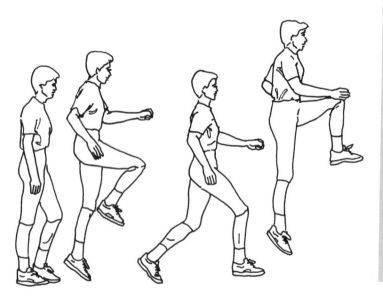

Equipment
None.

Start
Stand comfortably.

Action
Lift the right leg with the knee bent 90 degrees while lifting the left arm, with the elbows also bent 90 degrees. As these two limbs come back down, lift the opposite limbs with the same motion. For added difficulty, push off the ground for more upward extension.

Power Skipping

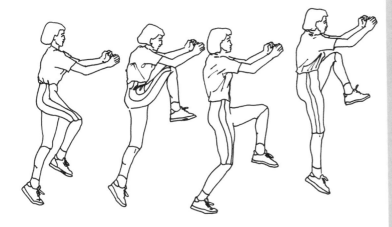

Equipment
None.

Start
Stand comfortably.

Action
Hold both arms out in front of you at shoulder height. Moving forward in a skipping motion, raise the leading knee to the chest, attempting to touch the foot with the hands. Repeat the motion with the opposite leg and continue skipping for the prescribed distance.

Backward Skipping

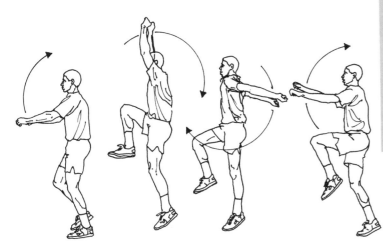

Equipment
A mark 20 to 30 meters from the start.

Start
Stand on one foot.

Action
Skip backward for 20 to 30 meters. Coordinate the arm swing with the skip to add to the backward propulsion.

Side Skipping With Big Arm Swing

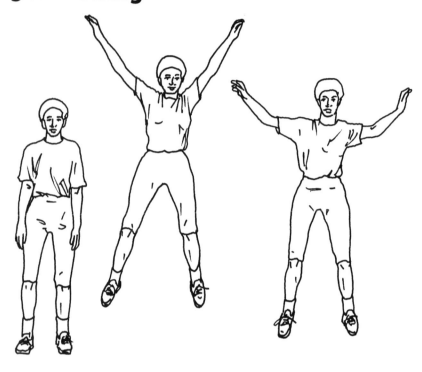

Moving Split Squat With Cycle

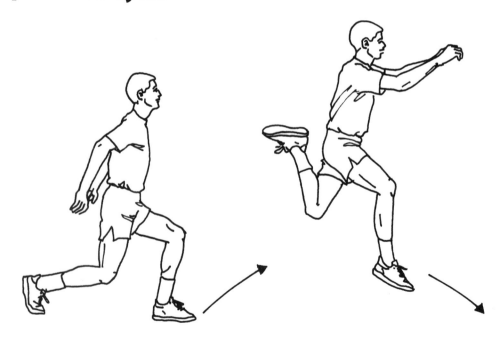

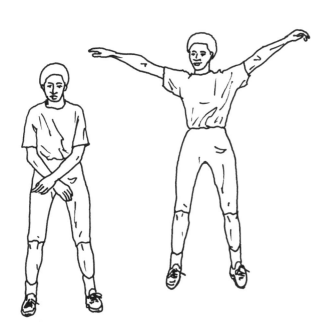

Equipment
None.

Start
Stand with feet together.

Action
This exercise looks like a jumping jack. Slide step to the side, swinging the arms up and over the head. As you push to bring the feet back together, the arms come back down and cross in front of the body. Keep performing this extended side step and arm swing for a prescribed distance (about 40 to 50 meters).

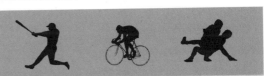

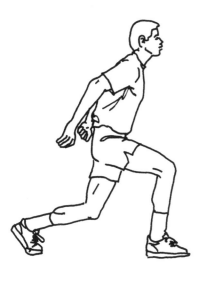

Equipment
A 30-meter mark.

Start
Spread the feet apart, front to back, and bend the front leg 90 degrees.

Action
Jumping up and forward, switch legs. As you bring the back leg through, try to touch the buttock. Land in the split-squat position and immediately do another cycle, continuing for a prescribed distance (about 30 meters). Each push from the ground has to propel the body forward. This is an advanced drill.

Alternate Bounding With Single Arm Action

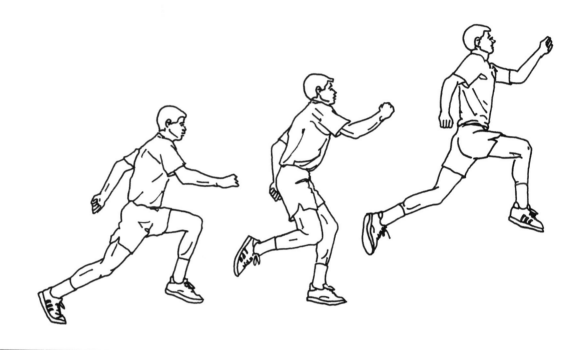

Alternate Bounding With Double Arm Action

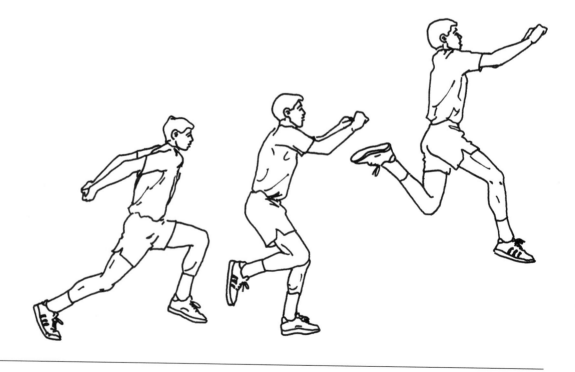

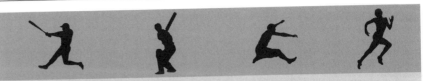

Equipment

None.

Start

Jog into the start of the drill to increase forward momentum. As you jog, start the drill with the right foot forward and the left foot back.

Action

This drill is simply an exaggerated running action. Push off with the left foot and bring the leg forward, with the knee bent and the thigh parallel to the ground. At the same time reach forward with the right arm. As the left leg comes through, the right leg extends back and remains extended for the duration of the push-off. Hold this extended stride for a brief time, then land on the left foot. The right leg then drives through to the front bent position, the left arm reaches forward, and the left leg extends back. Make each stride long, and try to cover as much distance as possible.

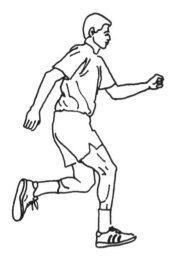

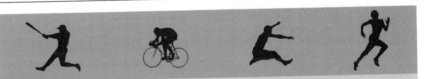

Equipment

None.

Start

Jog into the start of the drill to increase forward momentum. As you jog, start the drill with the right foot forward and the left foot back.

Action

Push off with the left foot and bring the leg forward, with the knee bent and the thigh parallel to the ground. At the same time bring both arms forward with great force to help propel the body forward. As the left leg comes through, the right leg extends back and remains extended for the duration of the push-off. Hold this extended stride for a brief time, quickly bring both arms behind the body, then land on the left foot. The right leg then drives through to the front bent position, the arms come forward, the left leg extends back, and the arms move back. This drill is an exaggerated running action; make each stride long, and try to cover as much distance as possible.

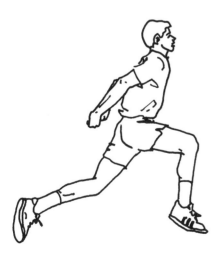

Combination Bounding With Single Arm Action

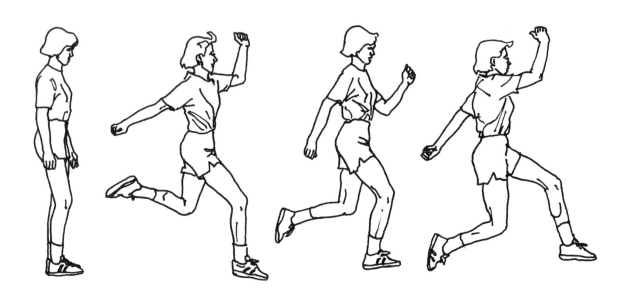

Combination Bounding With Double Arm Action

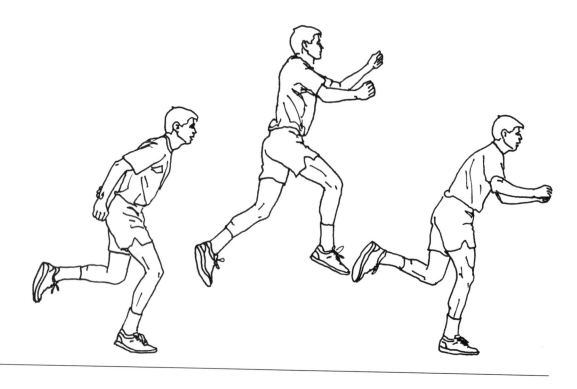

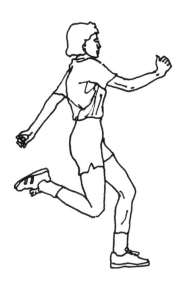

Equipment
None.

Start
Stand on one foot.

Action
In combination bounding you bound on one foot in a set sequence (right-right-left or left-left-right). Bound from one foot, then the same foot, then the other foot. The right arm moves forward with the left foot, and vice versa. Continue bounding by repeating the cycle.

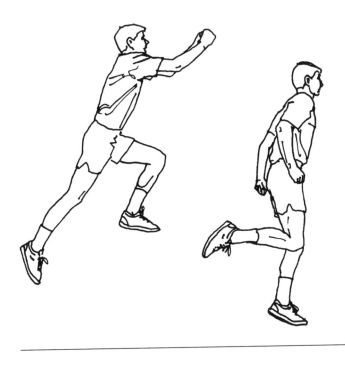

Equipment
None.

Start
Stand on one foot.

Action
In combination bounding you bound on one foot in a set sequence (right-right-left or left-left-right). Bound from one foot, then the same foot, then the other foot. Swing both arms forward on each bound, very quickly, to keep the body balanced and the motion of the bound smooth.

Combination Bounding With Vertical Jump

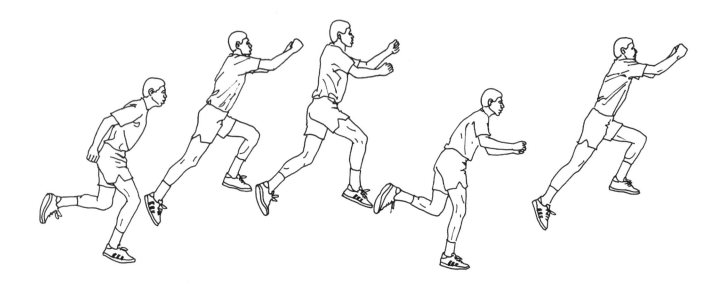

Single Leg Bounding

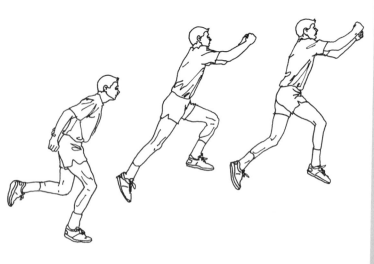

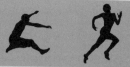

Equipment
None.

Start
Stand on one foot.

Action
Bound from one foot as far forward as possible, using the other leg and arms to cycle in the air for balance and to increase forward momentum. Advanced athletes should try to touch the heel of the bounding foot to the buttocks with each bound. Continue bounding for a prescribed distance (about 40 meters). This drill should be performed on both legs for equal strength.

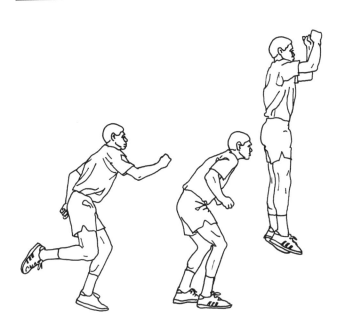

Equipment
None.

Start
Stand on one foot.

Action
Do a combination bounding sequence (right-right-left or left-left-right), then follow immediately with a strong vertical jump. On the third bound, bring the non-bounding foot up to meet the bounding foot so that the jump is off both feet. Use a double arm swing to assist in lifting you vertically. As soon as you land from the vertical jump, complete another bounding sequence.

TIP Think of the arm action during jumping as "punching." This will allow a maximal contribution to the overall height of the jump.

Medicine Ball Exercises

Front Toss	Low Post Drill
Heel Toss	Backward Throw
Over-Under	Backward Throw With Jump to Box
Trunk Rotation	Kneeling Side Throw
Underhand Throw	Quarter-Eagle Chest Pass
Pull-Over Pass	Medicine Ball Grab
Overhead Throw	Power Drop
Side Throw	Catch and Pass With Jump-and-Reach

TIP In theory, plyometrics for the upper extremities are no different than those for the lower extremities, so treat them the same. The exception is that you are working from a more mobile base with smaller muscles in the upper body. Elastic strength in the upper body and trunk is just as dependent upon stretching rapidly and using the recoil property of muscle as the legs.

Front Toss

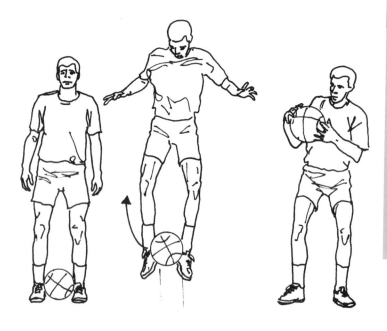

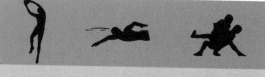

Equipment
A medicine ball.

Start
Stand with the ball held between your feet.

Action
Jump up with the ball, then with your legs toss it to yourself while in the air. After catching it, drop the ball to the ground between your feet and repeat.

Heel Toss

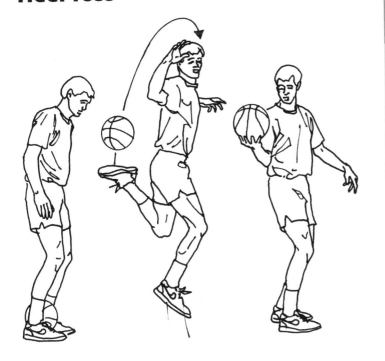

Equipment
A medicine ball.

Start
Stand with the ball held between your heels.

Action
Use the heel of one foot to flick the ball up and over your back and shoulders, and catch it in front of your body. This toss requires a quick flexion of the knee and considerable effort from the hamstring muscles.

Over-Under

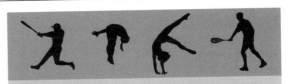

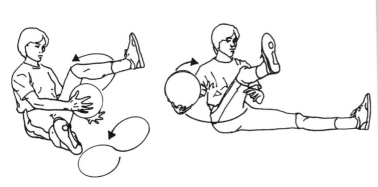

Equipment
A medicine ball.

Start
Sit on the floor with your legs and the ball straight in front of you.

Action
Lift your left leg and pass the ball under it from the inside. Then pass it over the top of your left leg, under your right leg from the inside, and over the top of your right leg (so the ball makes a figure eight around your legs).

Trunk Rotation

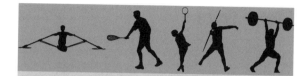

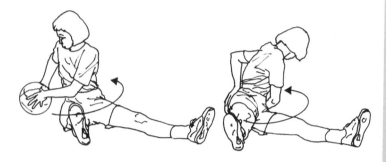

Equipment
A medicine ball.

Start
Sit on the floor with your legs spread and the ball behind your back.

Action
Rotate to the right, pick up the ball, bring it around to your left side, and replace it behind your back (so the ball makes a circle around your body). Repeat the prescribed number of times and then reverse directions.

Underhand Throw

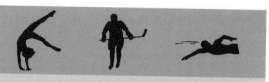

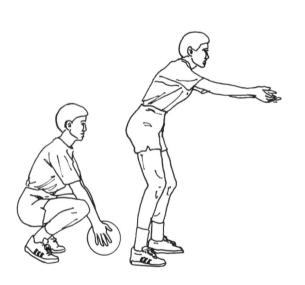

Equipment
A partner and a medicine ball.

Start
Stand in a squat holding the ball close to the ground about three meters from your partner.

Action
Keeping your back straight, raise straight up and throw the ball up and out to your partner, using the legs to provide momentum.

Pull-Over Pass

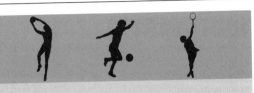

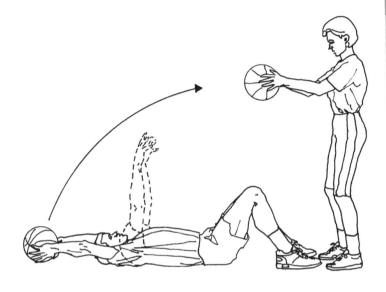

Equipment
A partner and a medicine ball.

Start
Lie on your back with your knees bent, holding the ball on the floor behind your head, while your partner stands at your feet.

Action
Keeping your arms extended, pass the ball to your partner. Your partner can back up to require you to throw farther for increased intensity.

Overhead Throw

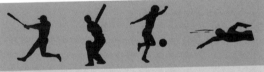

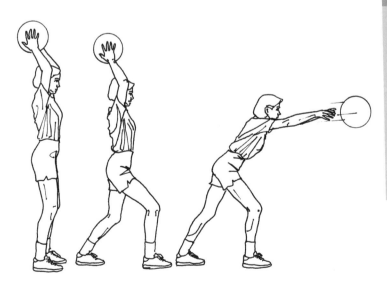

Equipment
A medicine ball and a partner.

Start
Stand with a medicine ball overhead.

Action
Step forward and bring the ball sharply forward with both arms throwing it to a partner or over a specific distance.

Side Throw

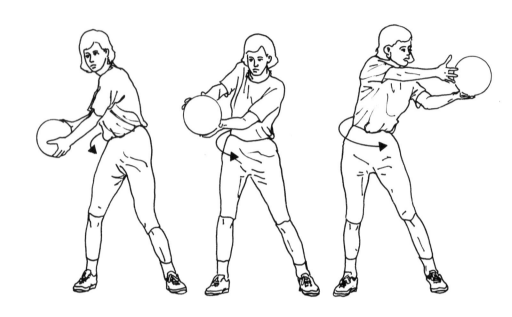

Low Post Drill

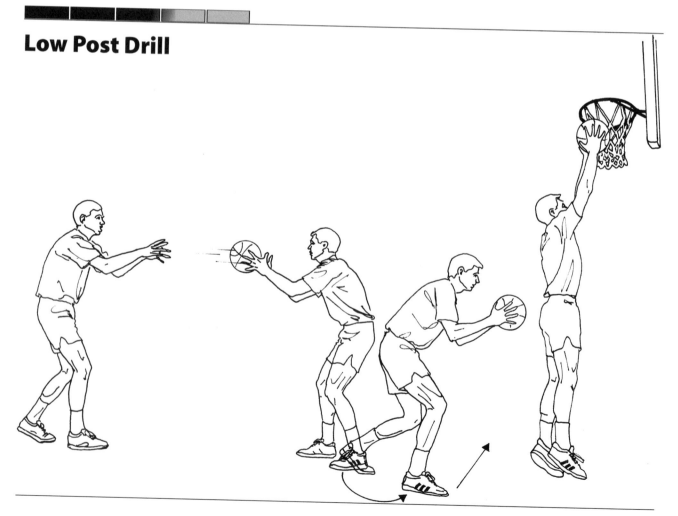

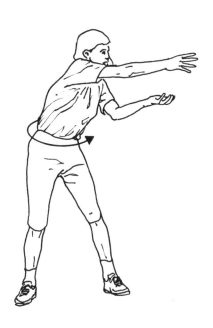

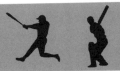

Equipment
A medicine ball and a partner or large solid barrier.

Start
Holding a medicine ball on your right, stand with feet shoulder-width apart.

Action
Swing the ball farther to the right and then forcefully reverse directions to the left and release. You may toss the ball to a partner or throw it against a solid barrier (e.g., a gym wall).

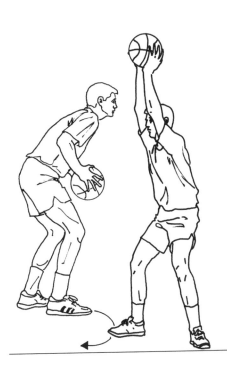

Equipment
A partner, a medicine ball, and a basketball goal.

Start
Stand with your back to the basket, about a meter to the front or side.

Action
Your partner starts the drill by throwing you the ball in the low post position. Catch it, pivot, and jump to touch the ball against the rim. Immediately after landing, jump to touch the rim with the ball a second time. Finally, pivot back toward your partner and pass the ball to him or her.

Backward Throw

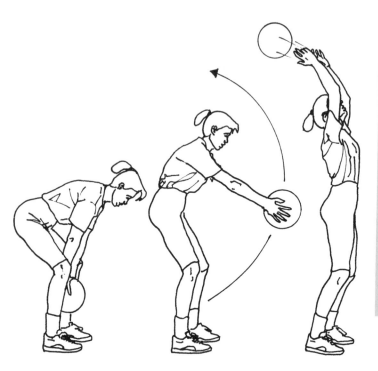

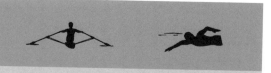

Equipment
A partner and a medicine ball.

Start
Stand about three meters in front of your partner, facing the same direction and holding the ball in front of you.

Action
Holding the ball between your legs, squat down and then toss the ball up and over your head to your partner. Be careful to bend your knees, bend from your hips, and keep your back straight.

Backward Throw With Jump to Box

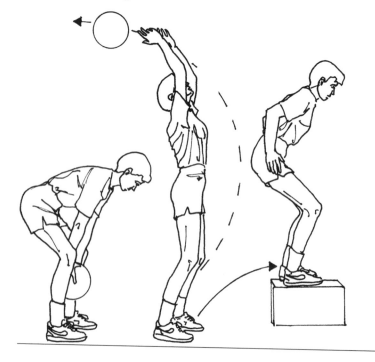

Equipment
A box 12 to 42 inches high and a medicine ball.

Start
Squat facing the box and holding a medicine ball.

Action
Lower the ball between your legs, then toss it up and back over your head. As you thrust upward to toss the ball, push off the ground and land on the box. Step off the box and collect the ball for the next repetition.

Kneeling Side Throw

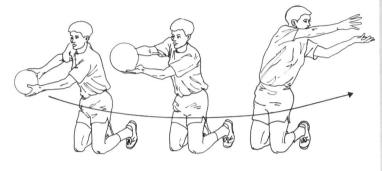

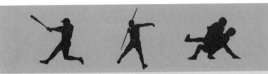

Equipment
A partner and a medicine ball.

Start
Kneel with your partner about three meters to the side and hold the ball to the other side with both hands at hip level.

Action
Twist your upper body and arms together and throw the ball to your partner.

Quarter-Eagle Chest Pass

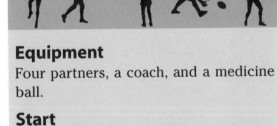

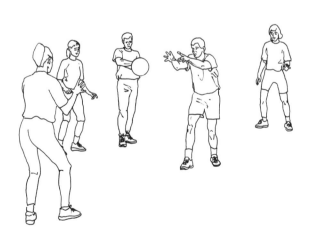

Equipment
Four partners, a coach, and a medicine ball.

Start
Assume a ready position with a partner in front of you, in back of you, and to each side.

Action
When the coach calls out "right" or "left," turn the body quickly a quarter turn and pass the ball to the person facing you. Drill continues for 10 to 12 passes.

Medicine Ball Grab

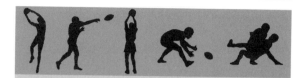

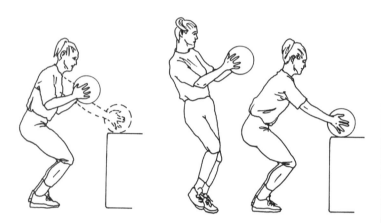

Equipment
10- to 25-pound medicine ball set up on a box 18 to 24 inches high.

Start
Stand in a "ready" position with the ball directly in front of you.

Action
On the "go" command, reach forward and grab the ball and drop back into the "ready" position as quickly as possible. In addition, you may pump the ball to the full extension of your arms for three to five repetitions after hitting the ready position.

Power Drop

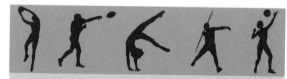

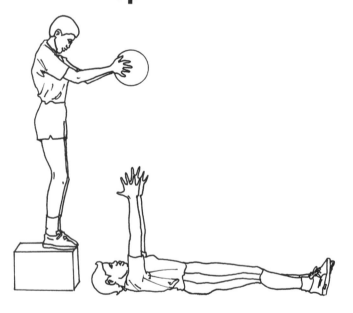

Equipment
A partner, a box 12 to 42 inches high, and a medicine ball.

Start
Lie supine on the ground with arms stretched upward over chest. Partner stands on the box holding the medicine ball at arm's length.

Action
Partner drops the ball. Catch the ball and immediately propel the ball back to the partner. Repeat.

Catch and Pass
With Jump-and-Reach

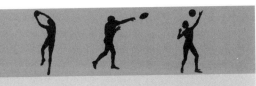

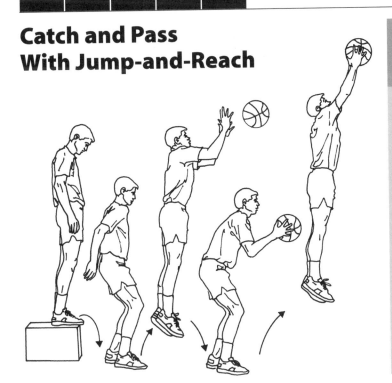

Equipment

A partner, a box 12 to 42 inches high, a medicine ball, and a high object (like a basketball goal).

Start

Stand on the box, feet shoulder-width apart and toes close to the edge.

Action

Step off the box and land on both feet. Explode up and forward, extend your arms, and catch a pass from your partner. Upon landing, explode up again and reach for the high object with the medicine ball.

SPORT-SPECIFIC DRILLS

This chapter shows you plyometric exercises that are most beneficial for each of 24 different sports or activities. An illustrated sequence of the exercise technique is shown, along with the name of the exercise and the page number on which the full explanation appears in chapter 4.

Jon Zuber: Minor League Baseball Player, Scranton/Wilkes-Barre Red Barons

Jon, an outfielder and first baseman for the Philadelphia Phillies' AAA club, presented a not-so-unique problem in that he showed up four weeks before he was to leave for baseball camp and wanted to try some specialized training. The opportunity for application of complex training was apparent. We decided to use specialized low-intensity plyometrics, running on a high-speed treadmill, and medicine ball work. He had been doing some work in the off-season and already had a good base of cardiovascular and strength training.

In complex training the idea is to perform a set of resistive exercises and follow it immediately with a set of plyometric exercises. The following is an example of a typical portion of his program:

3 sets of 10 reps back squats followed by 10 jumps to a box

3 sets of 10 reps lat pull-downs followed by 10 pull-over throws

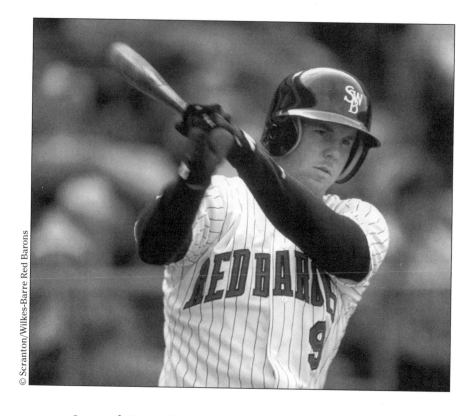

3 sets of 12 reps Russian twists followed by 12 side throws

3 sets of 12 reps alternate toe touches followed by 30 seconds of chinnies

2 sets of 15 reps side step-ups followed by 3 sets of the hexagon drill (3 times around each set)

This type of training is effective when attempting to get quick results in a short time frame. Since baseball spring training was so close, high-intensity and speed work were called for. Fortunately, Jon had a good base to work from and tolerated this type of training well.

Jon hit .315 in 1997, led his team with 37 doubles, and was named to the AAA All-Star team for the second consecutive year.

Baseball and Softball

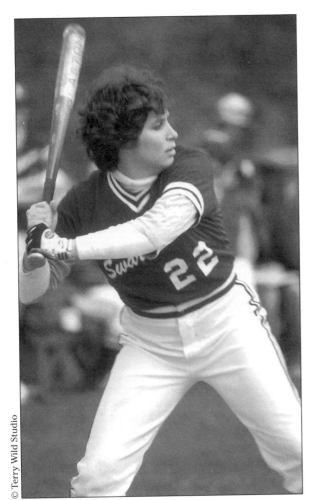

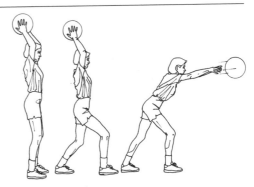

Overhead Throw (p. 135)

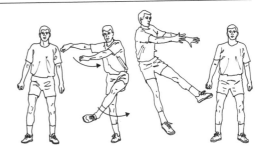

Lateral Jump With Two Feet (p. 88)

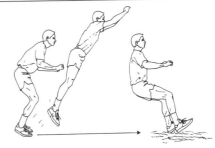

Standing Long Jump (p. 86)

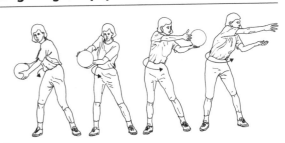

Side Throw (p. 136)

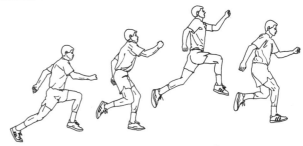

Alternate Bounding With Single Arm Action (p. 126)

Basketball

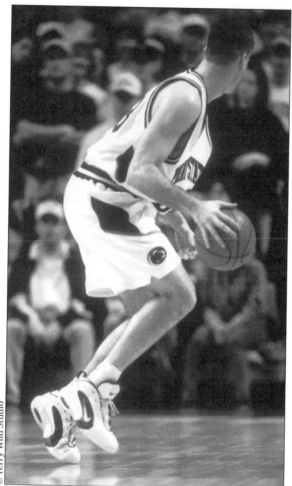

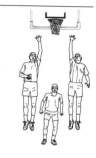

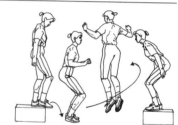

Rim Jumps (p. 96)

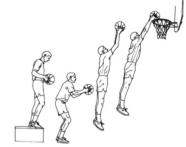

Depth Jump With Stuff (p. 118)

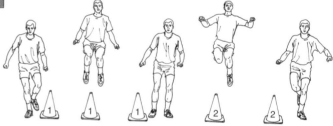

Depth Jump With 180-Degree Turn (p. 115)

Lateral Cone Hops (p. 98)

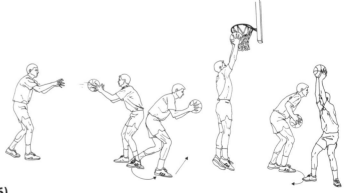

Low Post Drill (p. 136)

© Terry Wild Studio

Bicycling

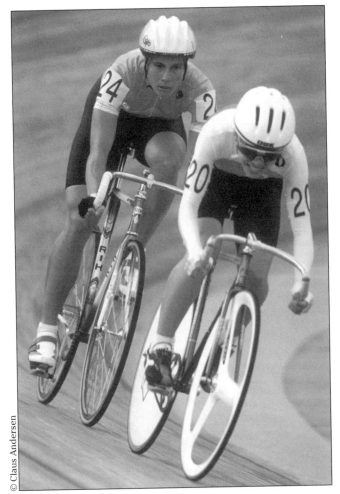

© Claus Andersen

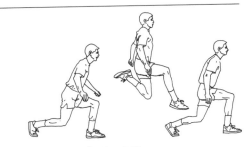

Split Squat With Cycle (p. 84)

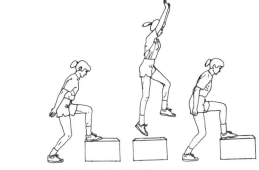

Single Leg Push-Off (p. 105)

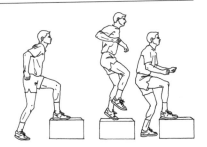

Alternating Push-Off (p. 104)

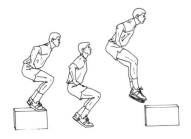

Squat Depth Jump (p. 114)

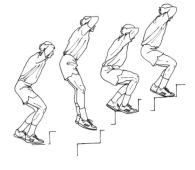

Stadium Hops (p. 100)

Cricket

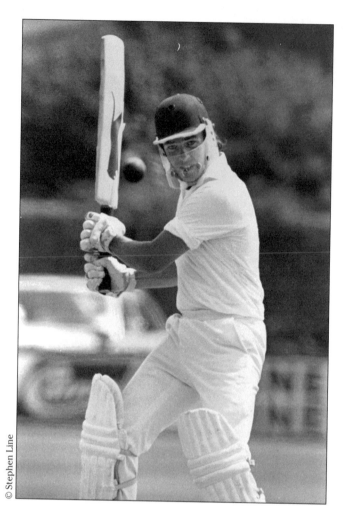

© Stephen Line

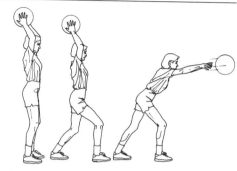

Overhead Throw (p. 135)

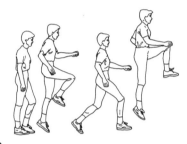

Skipping (p. 122)

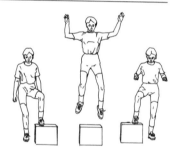

Side-to-Side Box Shuffle (p. 106)

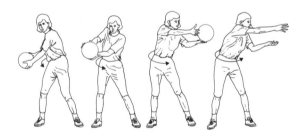

Side Throw (p. 136)

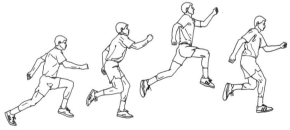

Alternate Bounding With Single Arm Action (p. 126)

Diving

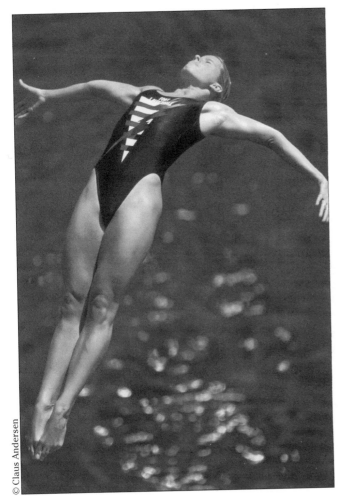

© Claus Andersen

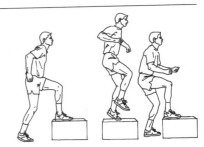

Alternating Push-Off (p. 104)

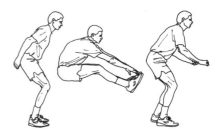

Straight Pike Jump (p. 85)

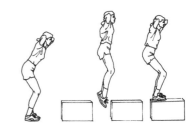

Front Box Jump (p. 106)

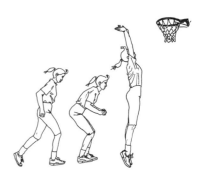

Step-Close Jump-and-Reach (p. 112)

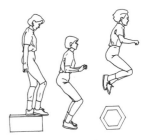

Depth Jump Over Barrier (p. 120)

Downhill Skiing

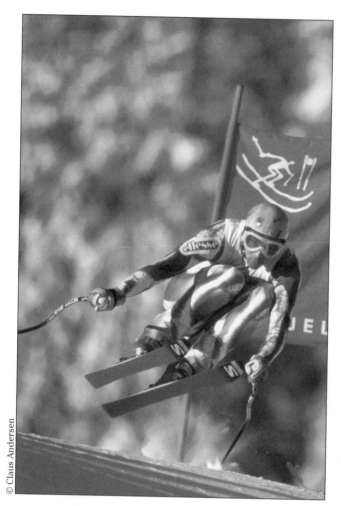

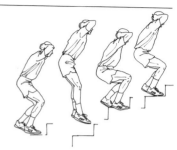

Stadium Hops (p. 100)

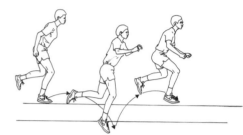

Zigzag Drill (p. 103)

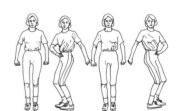

Hip-Twist Ankle Hop (p. 82)

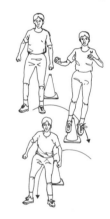

Diagonal Cone Hops (p. 95)

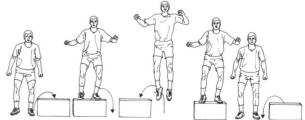

90-Second Box Drill (p. 108)

Figure Skating

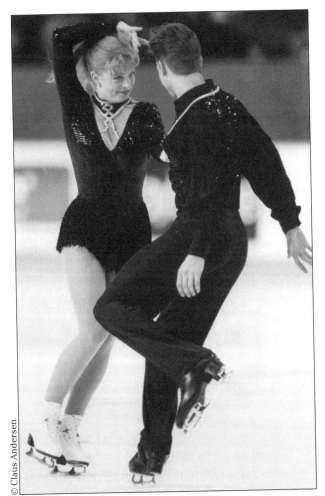

© Claus Andersen

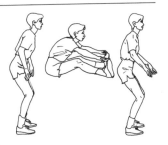

Split Pike Jump (p. 85)

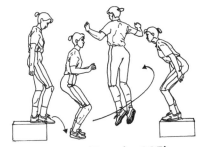

Depth Jump With 180-Degree Turn (p. 115)

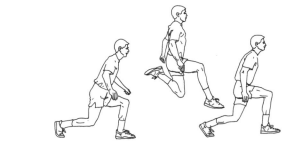

Split Squat With Cycle (p. 84)

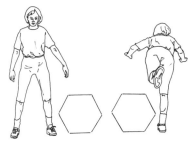

Straddle Jump to Camel Landing (p. 89)

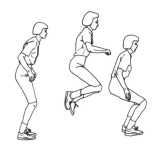

Double Leg Hops (p. 97)

Football

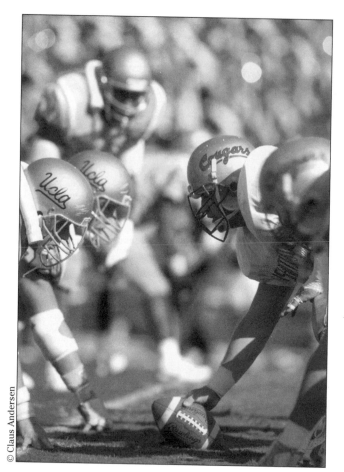

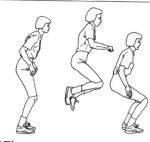

Double Leg Hops (p. 97)

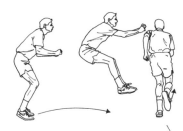

Standing Long Jump With Lateral Sprint (p. 89)

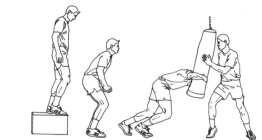

Depth Jump With Blocking Bag (p. 118)

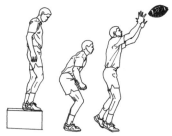

Depth Jump With Pass Catching (p. 119)

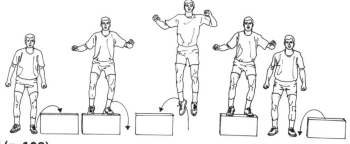

90-Second Box Drill (p. 108)

Gymnastics

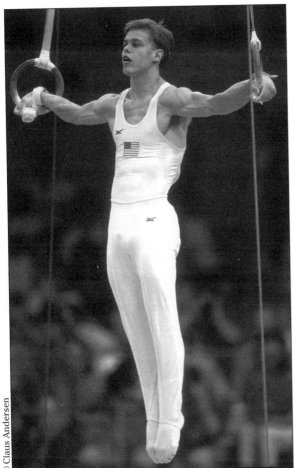

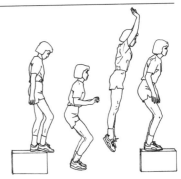

Depth Jump to Prescribed Height (p. 113)

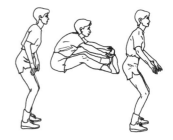

Split Pike Jump (p. 85)

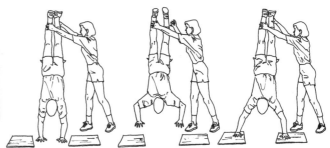

Handstand Depth Jump (p. 120)

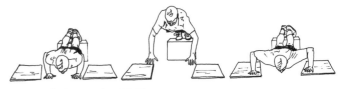

Incline Push-Up Depth Jump (p. 114)

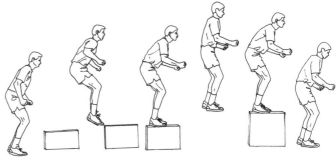

Pyramiding Box Hops (p. 108)

Ice Hockey

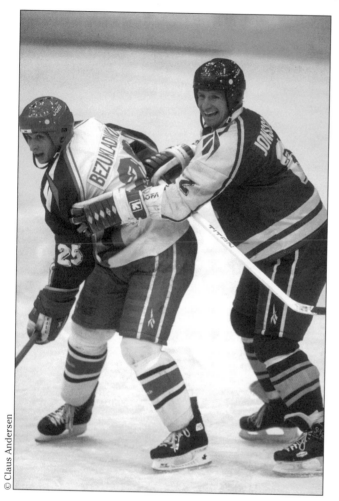

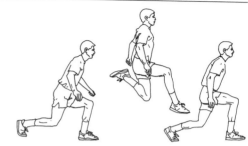

Split Squat With Cycle (p. 84)

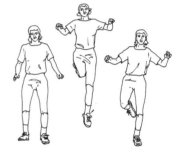

Lateral Jump With Single Leg (p. 90)

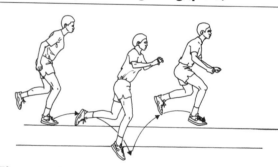

Zigzag Drill (p. 103)

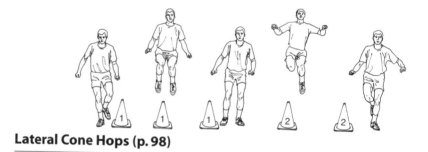

Lateral Cone Hops (p. 98)

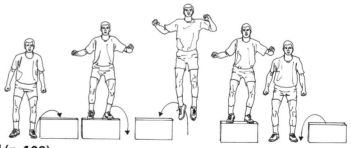

90-Second Box Drill (p. 108)

© Claus Andersen

In-Line/Speed Skating

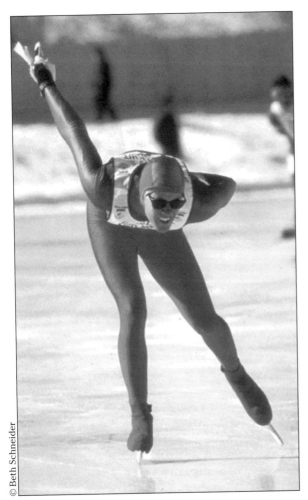

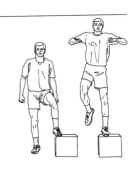

Lateral Step-Up (p. 105)

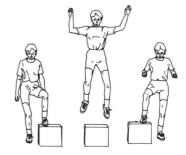

Side-to-Side Box Shuffle (p. 106)

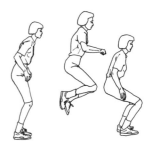

Double Leg Hops (p. 97)

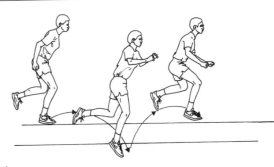

Zigzag Drill (p. 103)

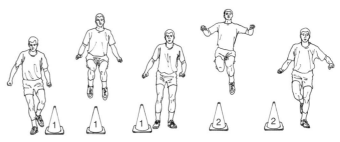

Lateral Cone Hops (p. 98)

Netball

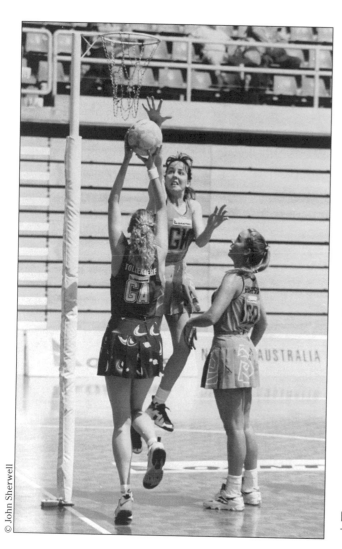

© John Sherwell

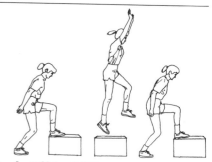

Single Leg Push-Off (p. 105)

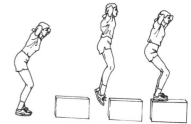

Front Box Jump (p. 106)

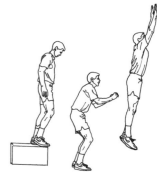

Depth Jump (p. 113)

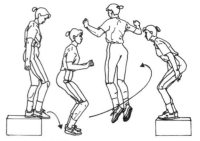

Depth Jump With 180-Degree Turn (p. 115)

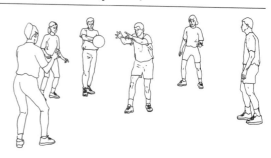

Quarter-Eagle Chest Pass (p. 139)

Rowing

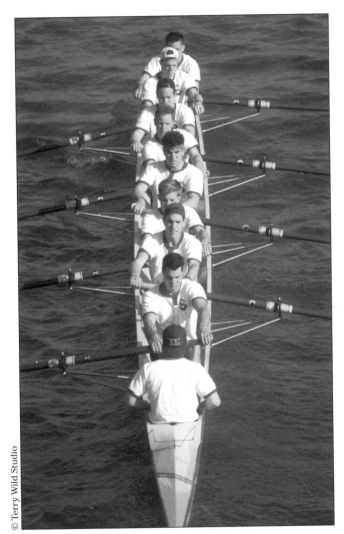

© Terry Wild Studio

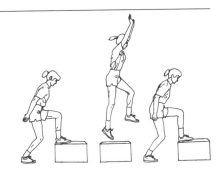

Single Leg Push-Off (p. 105)

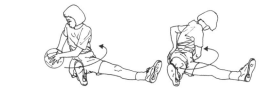

Multiple Box-to-Box Squat Jumps (p. 110)

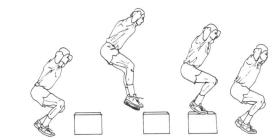

Trunk Rotation (p. 134)

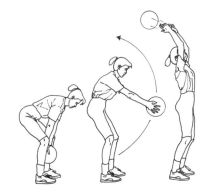

Backward Throw (p. 138)

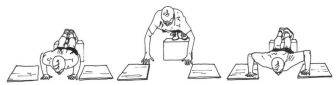

Incline Push-Up Depth Jump (p. 114)

Rugby

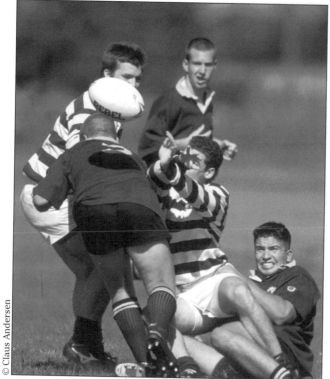

© Claus Andersen

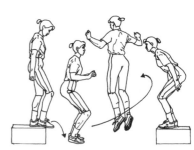

Depth Jump With 180- and 360-Degree Turn (p. 115, 116)

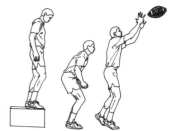

Depth Jump With Pass Catching (p. 119)

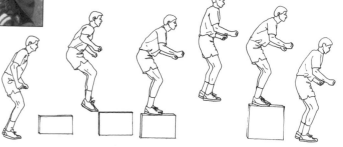

Pyramiding Box Hops (p. 108)

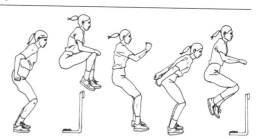

Barrier Hops (Hurdle Hops) (p. 98)

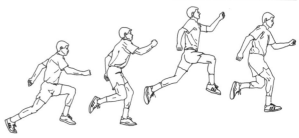

Alternate Bounding With Single Arm Action (p. 126)

Soccer

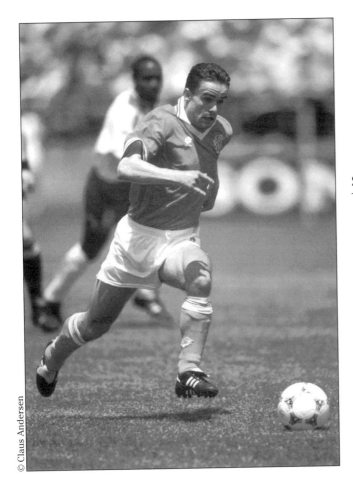

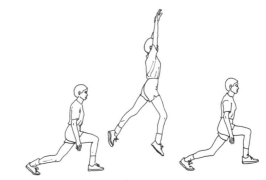

Split Squat Jump (p. 83)

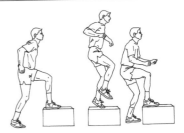

Lateral Jump Over Barrier (p. 90)

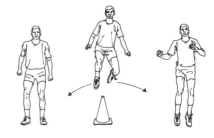

Alternating Push-Off (p. 104)

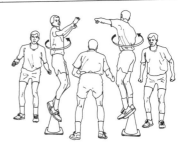

Cone Hops With 180-Degree Turn (p. 97)

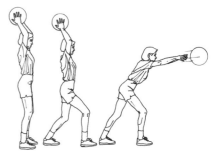

Overhead Throw (p. 135)

© Claus Andersen

Squash/Racquetball

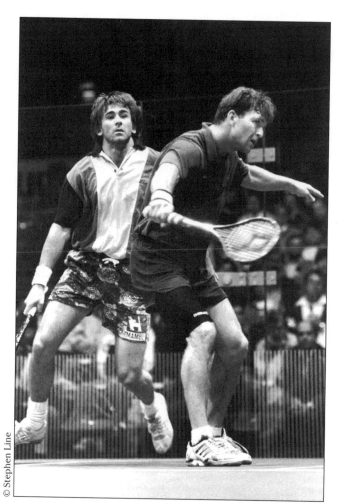

© Stephen Line

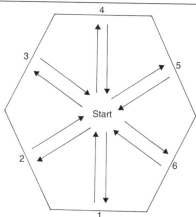

Hexagon Drill (p. 94)

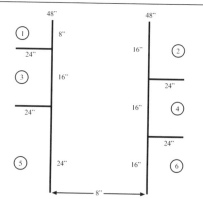

Munoz Formation (p. 75)

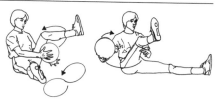

Over-Under (p. 133)

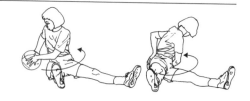

Trunk Rotation (p. 134)

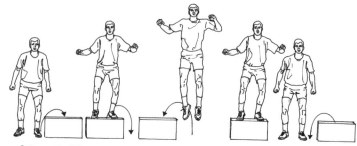

30-, 60-, or 90-Second Box Drill (p. 108)

Swimming

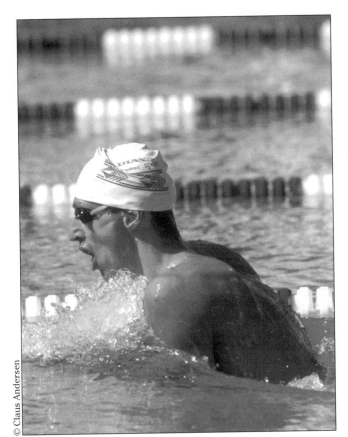

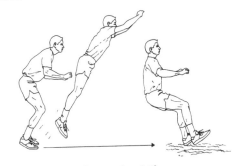

Standing Long Jump (p. 86)

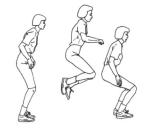

Double Leg Hops (p. 97)

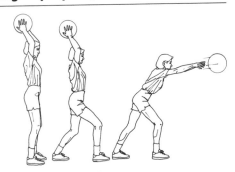

Overhead Throw (p. 135)

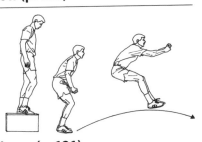

Depth Jump to Standing Long Jump (p. 121)

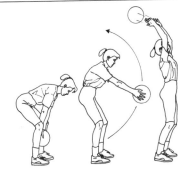

Backward Throw (p. 138)

© Claus Andersen

Tennis

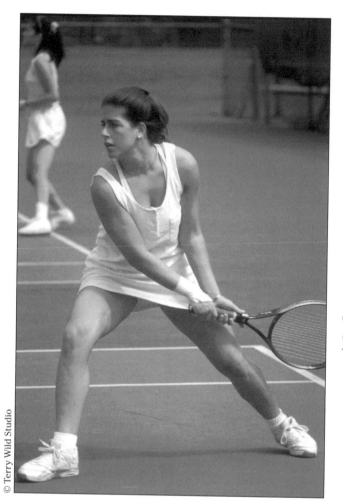

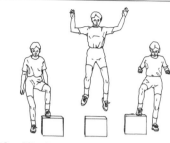

Side-to-Side Box Shuffle (p. 106)

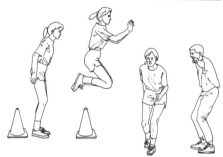

Cone Hops With Change of Direction Sprint (p. 96)

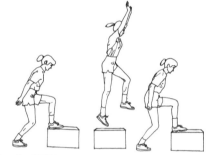

Single Leg Push-Off (p. 105)

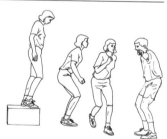

Depth Jump With Lateral Movement (p. 117)

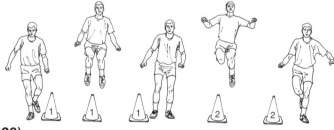

Lateral Cone Hops (p. 98)

Track and Field: Jumping Events

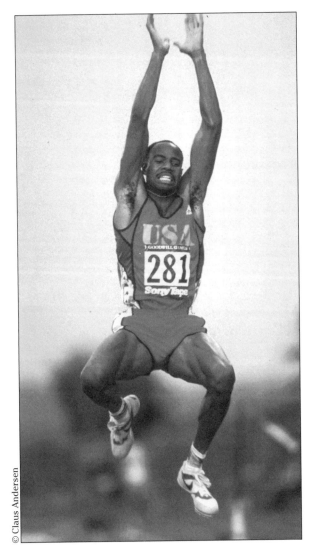

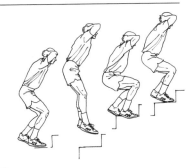

Stadium Hops (p. 100)

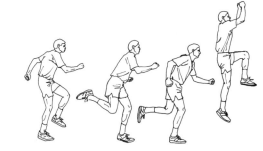

Single Leg Bounding (p. 130)

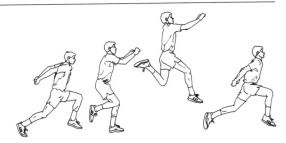

1-2-3 Drill (p. 88)

Alternate Bounding With Double Arm Action (p. 126)

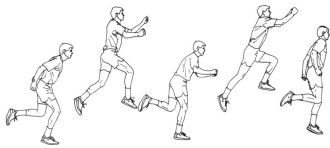

Combination Bounding With Double Arm Action (p. 128)

Track and Field: Sprints

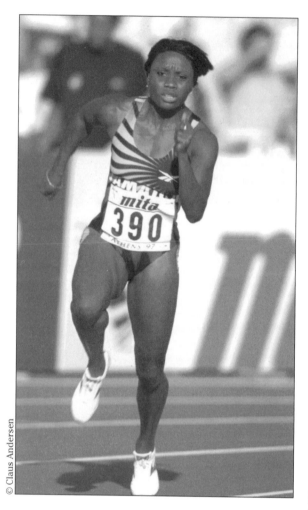

© Claus Andersen

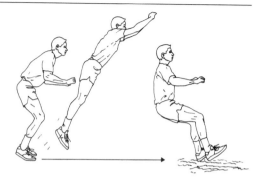

Standing Long Jump (p. 86)

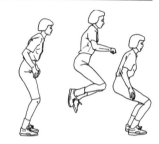

Double Leg Hops (p. 97)

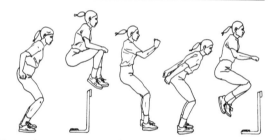

Barrier Hops (Hurdle Hops) (p. 98)

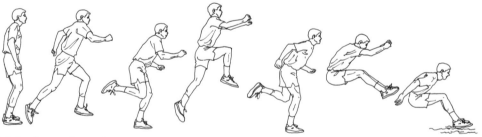

Standing Triple Jump (p. 92)

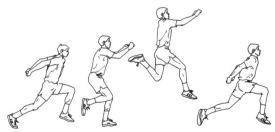

Alternate Bounding With Double Arm Action (p. 126)

Track and Field: Throwing Events

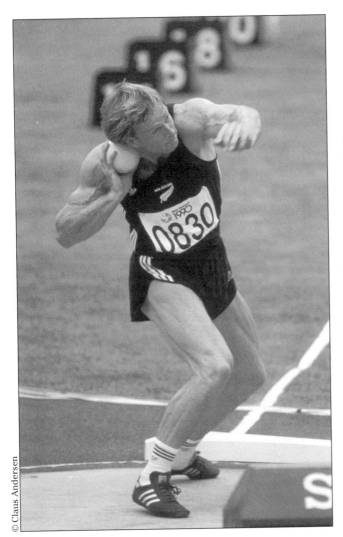

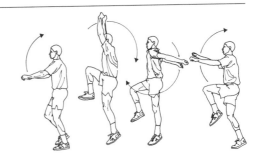

Backward Skipping (p. 123)

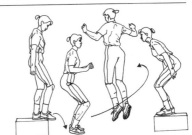

Backward Throw With Jump to Box (p. 138)

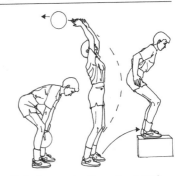

Depth Jump With 180-Degree Turn (p. 115)

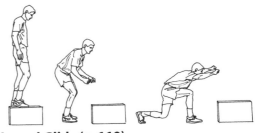

Depth Jump With Backward Glide (p. 119)

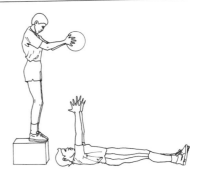

Power Drop (p. 140)

© Claus Andersen

Volleyball

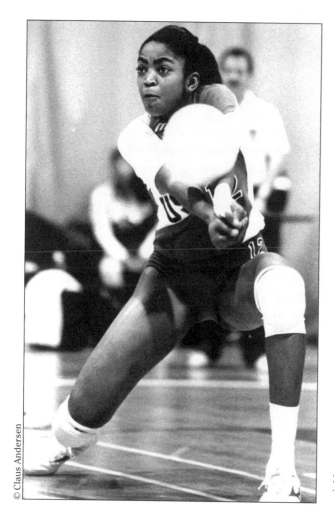

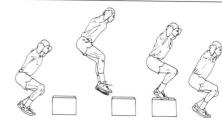

Multiple Box-to-Box Squat Jumps (p. 110)

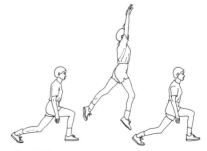

Depth Jump (p. 113)

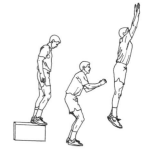

Split Squat Jump (p. 83)

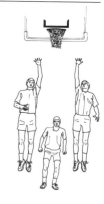

Rim Jumps (p. 96)

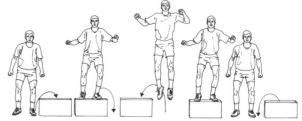

90-Second Box Drill (p. 108)

Weightlifting

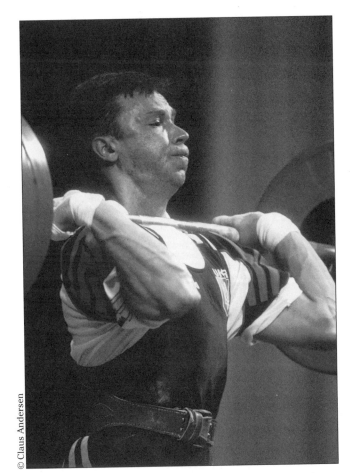

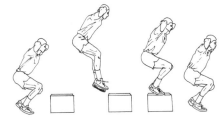

Split Squat Jump (p. 83)

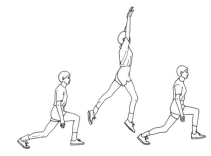

Multiple Box-to-Box Squat Jumps (p. 110)

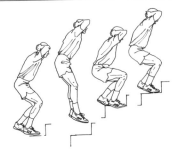

Stadium Hops (p. 100)

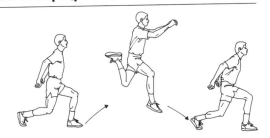

Moving Split Squat With Cycle (p. 124)

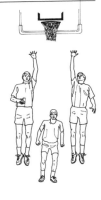

Rim Jumps (p. 96)

Wrestling

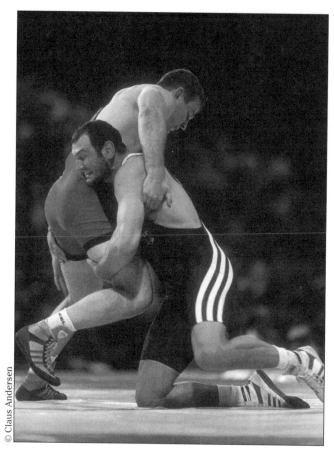

© Claus Andersen

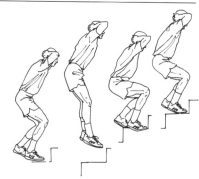

Stadium Hops (p. 100)

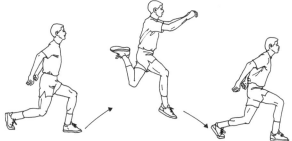

Moving Split Squat With Cycle (p. 124)

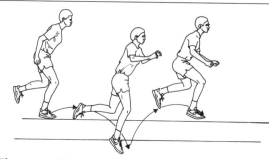

Zigzag Drill (p. 103)

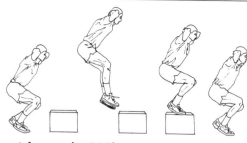

Multiple Box-to-Box Squat Jumps (p. 110)

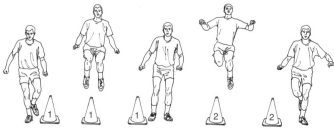

Lateral Cone Hops (p. 98)

BIBLIOGRAPHY

Adams, K., O'Shea, J., O'Shea, K., & Climstein, M. (1992). The effect of six weeks of squat, plyometric and squat-plyometric training on power production. *Journal of Applied Sports Science Research*, 6(1), 36-41.

Adams, T. (1984). An investigation of selected plyometric training exercises on muscular leg strength and power. *Track and Field Quarterly Review*, 84(1), 36-40.

Allerheiligen, B., & Rogers, R. (1995). Plyometrics program design. *Journal of Strength and Conditioning*, 17(4), 26-31.

Asmussen, E., & Bonde-Peterson, F. (1974). Storage of elastic energy in skeletal muscles in man. *Acta Physiologica Scandinavica*, 91, 385-392.

Auferoth, S. (1986). Power training for the developing thrower. *National Strength Coaches Association Journal*, 8(5), 56-62.

Bielik, E., Chu, D., & Costello, F., et al. (1986). Round-table: Practical considerations for utilizing plyometrics, part 1. *National Strength Coaches Association Journal*, 8(3), 14-22.

Bielik, E., Chu, D., & Costello, F., et al. (1986). Round-table: Practical considerations for utilizing plyometrics, part 2. *National Strength Coaches Association Journal*, 8(4), 14-24.

Blattner, S., & Noble, L. (1979). Relative effects of isokinetic and plyometric training on vertical jumping performance. *Research Quarterly*, 50(4), 583-588.

Bosco, C. (1982). Physiological considerations on vertical jump exercise after drops from variable heights. *Volleyball Technical Journal*, 6, 53-58.

Bosco, C., & Komi, P. (1979). Potentiation of the mechanical behavior of the human skeletal muscle through prestretching. *Acta Physiologica Scandinavica*, 106, 467-472.

Bosco, C., Komi, P., Pulli, P., Pittera, C., & Montoneu, J. (1982). Considerations of the training of the elastic potential of the human skeletal muscle. *Volleyball Technical Journal*, 6, 75-81.

Bosco, C., Luhtanen, P., & Komi, P. (1976). Kinetics and kinematics of the takeoff in the long jump. In P. Komi (Ed.), *Biomechanics VB* (pp. 174-180). Baltimore: University Park Press.

Brant, J. (1988, September). I'd like to explode. *Outside Magazine*, pp. 29-31.

Brown, M., Mayhew, J., & Boleach, L. (1986). The effect of plyometric training on the vertical jump of high school boys' basketball players. *Journal of Sports Medicine and Physical Fitness*, 26(1), 1-4.

Cavagna, G. (1970). Elastic bounce of the body. *Journal of Applied Physiology,* 29(3), 279-282.

Chu, D. (1983). Plyometrics: The link between strength and speed. *National Strength Coaches Association Journal,* 5(2), 20-21.

Chu, D. (1984). The language of plyometrics. *National Strength Coaches Association Journal,* 6(4), 30-31.

Chu, D. (1984). Plyometric exercise. *National Strength Coaches Association Journal,* 6(5), 56-62.

Chu, D. (1989). *Plyometric Exercises With the Medicine Ball.* Livermore, CA: Bittersweet.

Chu, D. (1996). *Explosive power and strength.* Champaign, IL: Human Kinetics.

Costello, F. (1984). *Bounding to the top.* Los Altos, CA: Tafnew.

Drez, D., Paine, R., & Roberts, T. (1987). *Abstract: Functional testing of 50 high school football players.* Unpublished study.

Duda, M. (1988). Plyometrics: A legitimate form of power training? *The Physician and Sportsmedicine Journal,* 16(3), 218.

Dursenev, L., & Raeysky, L. (1979). Strength training for jumpers. *Soviet Sports Review,* 14(2), 53-55.

Dyatchkov, V. (1969). High jumping, track technique. *Journal of Technical Track and Field Athletics,* 36, 1123-1158.

Frappier, J. (1995). *Acceleration Program training manual.* Fargo, ND: Acceleration Products, Inc.

Gambetta, V. (1978). Plyometric training. *USTCA Quarterly Review,* 2, 58-59.

Gehri, D., Ricard, M., Kleiner, D., Kirkendall, D. (n.d.). A comparison of plyometric training techniques for improving vertical jumping ability and energy production. *Strength and Conditioning.* Forthcoming.

Grieve, D. (1970). Stretching active muscles. *Track Technique,* 42, 1333-1335.

Harman, E., Rosenstein, M., Frykman, P., & Rosenstein, R. (1991). The effects of arms and countermovement on vertical jumping. *National Strength & Conditioning Journal,* 13(2), 38-39.

Holcomb, W., Lander, J., Rutland, R., & Wilson, G. (1996). A biomechanical analysis of the vertical jump and three modified plyometric depth jumps. *Journal of Strength and Conditioning Research,* 10(2), 83-88.

Holcomb, W., Lander, J., Rutland, R., & Wilson, G. (1996). The effectiveness of a modified plyometric program on power and the vertical jump. *Journal of Strength and Conditioning Research,* 10(2), 89-92.

Huber, J. (1987). Increasing a diver's vertical jump through plyometric training. *National Strength Coaches Association Journal,* 9(1), 34-36.

Komi, P. (1979). Neuromuscular performance: Factors influencing force and speed production. *Scandinavian Journal of Sports Science,* 1, 2-15.

Komi, P., & Bosco, C. (1978). Utilization of stored elastic energy in leg extensor muscles by men and women. *Medicine and Science in Sports and Exercise,* 10(4), 261-265.

Komi, P., & Buskirk, E. (1972). Effect of eccentric and concentric muscle conditioning on tension and electrical activity of human muscle. *Ergonomics*, 15, 417-434.

Lundin, P. (1985). A review of plyometric training. *National Strength Coaches Association Journal*, 7(69), 69-74.

Lyttle, A., Wilson, G., & Ostrowski, K. (1996). Enhancing performance: Maximal power versus combined weights and plyometrics training. *Journal of Strength and Conditioning Research*, 10(3), 173-179.

Matveyey, L. (1977). *Fundamentals of sports training*. Moscow: Progress Publishers.

McFarlane, B. (1983). Special strength: Horizontal and/or vertical? *Track and Field Quarterly Review*, 83(4), 51-53.

Miller, J. (1981). Plyometric training for speed. *National Strength Coaches Association Journal*, 2(3), 20-22.

Newton, R., & Kraemer, W. (1994). Developing explosive muscular power: Implications for a mixed methods training strategy. *National Strength and Conditioning Journal*, 16(5), 20-31.

Plisk, S. (1988). Physiological training for competitive alpine skiing. *National Strength Coaches Association Journal*, 10(1), 30-33.

Polhemus, R. (1980). The effects of plyometric training with ankle and vest weights on conventional weight programs for men. *Texas Coach*, 16-17.

Polhemus, R. (1980, February). The effects of plyometric training with ankle and vest weights on conventional weight programs for women. *Texas Coach*, 16-18.

Polhemus, R., & Burkhardt, E. (1980, March). The effects of plyometric training drills on the physical strength gains of collegiate football players. *National Strength Coaches Association Journal*, 2(1), 13-15.

Rasulbekov, R., Fomin, R., Chulkov, V., & Chudovsky, V. (1986). Does a swimmer need explosive strength? *National Strength Coaches Association Journal*, 8(2), 56-57.

Scoles, G. (1978). Depth jumping! Does it really work? *Athletic Journal*, 58, 48-75.

Stone, M., & O'Bryant, H. (1987). *Weight training: A scientific approach*. Edina, MN: Burgess International Group.

Verhoshanski, V. (1967). Are depth jumps useful? *Track and Field*, 12, 9.

Verhoshanski, V. (1969). Perspectives in the improvement of speed-strength preparation of jumpers. *Review of Soviet Physical Education and Sports*, 4(2), 28-29.

Verhoshanski, V., & Chernovsov, G. (1974). Jumps in the training of a sprinter. *Track and Field*, 9, 16-17.

Verhoshanski, V., & Tatyan, V. (1983). Speed-strength preparation of future champions. *Soviet Sports Review*, 18(4), 166-170.

Vermeil, A. (1989). Game day inseason training for the Chicago Bulls. *National Strength Coaches Association Journal*, 11(1), 47-48.

Vermeil, A. (1996). Personal communication.

Vermeil, A., & Chu, D. (1982). Periodization of strength training for professional football. *National Strength Coaches Association Journal*, 4(3), 54-55.

Vermeil, A., & Chu, D. (1983). A theoretical approach to planning a football season. *National Strength Coaches Association Journal*, 4(6), 33-36.

Wilt, F. (1975). Plyometrics—What it is and how it works. *Athletic Journal*, 55(5), 76, 89-90.

Worlick, M. (1983). Power development through plyometric exercise. *Soccer Journal*, 27, 39-41.

Yessis, M. (1982). Soviet conditioning for American football. *National Strength Coaches Association Journal*, 4(1), 4-7.

Young, W., Pryor, J., & Wilson, G. (1995). Effect of instructions on characteristics of countermovement and drop jump performance. *Journal of Strength and Conditioning Research*, 9(4), 232-236.

INDEX

ABOUT THE AUTHOR

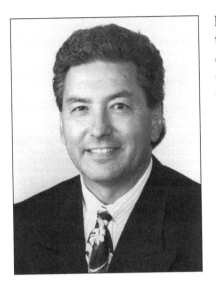

Dr. Donald Chu is a leading authority on power training and conditioning. He has been a conditioning consultant for the Chicago Bulls, Golden State Warriors, Milwaukee Bucks, Detroit Lions, and Chicago White Sox as well as for the United States Tennis Association and the 1996 U.S. Olympic synchronized swimming team, which took home the gold medal. He is the owner and director of NovaCare Clinic in Castro Valley, California, where he acts as a consultant to individual athletes.

Dr. Chu is president of the National Strength and Conditioning Association (NSCA). He is a licensed physical therapist, a certified athletic trainer through the National Athletic Trainers' Association (NATA), and a certified strength and conditioning specialist through the NSCA. He has received many honors, including the 1998 Dr. Ernst Jokl Sports Medicine Award, presented by the board of trustees of the United States Sports Academy; the 1995 NATA Most Distinguished Athletic Trainer Award; and the 1993 NSCA President's Award for Service. In 1978, his only year as a head coach, Dr. Chu was named the Far Western Conference Track and Field Coach of the Year.

Dr. Chu, who earned a PhD in physical therapy and kinesiology from Stanford University, is the program director for the physical therapist assistant program at Ohlone College in Fremont, California. He is also a professor emeritus of kinesiology and physical education at California State University, Hayward. He lives in Alameda, California.

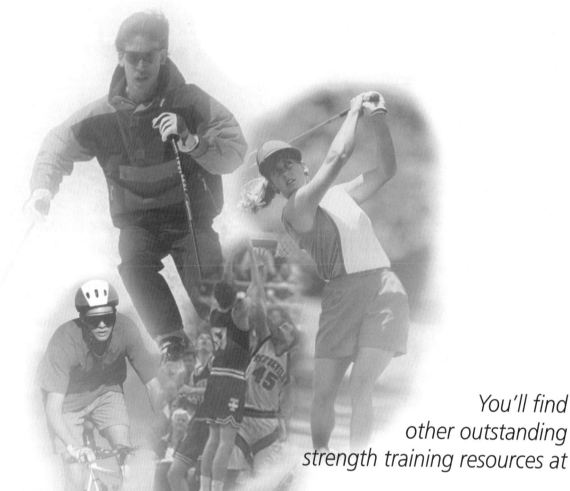